OPEN HEART SURGERY

A Second Chance

Nyles V. Reinfeld

With an Introduction By
William P. Sheldon, Chief Cardiologist
Cleveland Clinic Foundation

And Special Comments By
Alexander P. Ormond, Jr., Cardiologist
William E. Moats, M.D. and James F. Grow, Jr., M.D.

and

Danni Gogol Nadler, R.N.

and

The Reverend Dr. David H. Burnham

Prentice-Hall, Inc., Englewood Cliffs, NJ 07632

Library of Congress Cataloging in Publication Data

REINFELD, NYLES V. (date)
  Open heart surgery.

  Includes index.
    1. Heart—Surgery. 2. Heart—Surgery—Patients—
United States—Biography. 3. Reinfeld, Nyles V.
I. Ormond, Alexander P. II. Title. [DNLM: 1. Heart
surgery—Personal narratives. WG 169 R367o]
RD598.R45 1983   617'.412   83-3127
ISBN 0-13-637520-0
ISBN 0-13-637512-X (pbk.)

Editorial/production supervision: **Karen Skrable**
Interior design: **Karen Skrable and Rosalie Herion**
Manufacturing buyer: **Anthony Caruso**
Cover design: **Ben Santora**

Printed in the United States of America

10 9 8 7 6 5 4 3 2 1

ISBN 0-13-637520-0
ISBN 0-13-637512-X {PBK.}

Prentice-Hall International, Inc., *London*
Prentice-Hall of Australia Pty. Limited, *Sydney*
Editora Prentice-Hall do Brasil, Ltda., *Rio de Janeiro*
Prentice-Hall Canada Inc., *Toronto*
Prentice-Hall of India Private Limited, *New Delhi*
Prentice-Hall of Japan, Inc., *Tokyo*
Prentice-Hall of Southeast Asia Pte. Ltd., *Singapore*
Whitehall Books Limited, *Wellington, New Zealand*

TO AN EIGHT-YEAR-OLD BOY

He never really knew, but he sensed and understood that his father lay seriously ill with a heart problem. They were alone in the house. The mother and daughters were out, and he was the man of the house. He watched TV for a while, then lay down on the floor beside the cot, put his feet up next to his father, and gripped his father's hand. After a while he got up. "Do you want to see me stand on my head?" he asked. "I'm getting better." He did this twice, then told me about the TV show he had seen. I nodded but was too sick to listen.

"Can I get you something?" he asked. "Water," I said. "With ice in it?" he asked. He left and in a few minutes returned, put a coaster under the glass, and set it on the floor next to me. He sat down, leaned against the cot, and waited quietly for the others to come home. He understood and cared.

To my son Nick—

Written March 5, 1975, just before my first heart operation.

OTHER BOOKS BY THE AUTHOR

Survival Management for Industry
Production and Inventory Control
Production Control
Mathematical Programming
      (co-authored with W.R. Vogel)

CONTENTS

PREFACE

In the past decade and a half, a miracle has been wrought. Thousands of people who might have died, or been bed-ridden, or suffered major restrictions in activity are moving about with a freedom only hoped for before the Korean War. In addition, those early operations, which were new miracles each time they were wrought, have become almost routine, following a chain of advances in practice, technique, and knowledge. The chances of success and the results have kept pace. Persons like myself, who had an early operation and then later needed a second, will probably skip this sequence completely, because so much has been learned in such a short time.

Situations that were at one time too serious to be considered for surgery are now handled effectively, giving hope not only to those who have suffered their first heart problems, but to those who are even less fortunate and have lived with a history of heart disease and heart-ache.

The annual number of operations today exceeds 100,000, so that the success ratio is clearly established. Some of the best known names in society, including Henry Kissinger, Rock Hudson, Raymond Firestone, Sen. Barry Goldwater, and the King of Saudi Arabia, have faced open heart surgery and returned to live a normal life.

Many of these men (and women) are as active today as they have been at any time in their lives. Harvey Kuenn, manager of the Milwaukee Brewers, won the American League Pennant in 1982, after his operations. The man's indomitable courage showed through every time he walked to the mound—on an artificial leg which was hardly discernible to the TV audience.

Your future has not necessarily been destroyed, as may now seem to be the case, but only interrupted. In fact as you learn to live with your problem, you may also be able to live more effectively.

But telling you these things is hardly enough to wipe away the anxieties. Open heart surgery, or any surgery, is not exactly something we look forward to. The threat is ominous; but then so is crossing the street. The latter we do all the time, and, as we get older and more preoccupied, we step out into the traffic without looking. We couldn't hear a horn if it were stuck in our ear. We survive against insurmountable odds because we trust some stranger, who may be drunk as a fish at the time, behind the wheel of a thundering behemoth. But this doesn't keep us from crossing the street, time after time, in our own inimitable manner.

The purpose of this book, however, is not to supply you with pollyannaish drivel. Rather, it is hoped that it will give you and your family a better understanding of what you face and how you feel about it. We all have fears that we cannot express. We all wonder about our future and worry about our responsibilities to our family. We feel guilty about our problem and wonder what we've done wrong. We suffer frustration and anger and emotional stress. In addition, we want to know more about the procedures that will be used. Finally, we want to know what will happen to us after it's over and we leave the hospital.

Most of these things have not been covered, heretofore, in the literature except piecemeal, and usually in an impersonal manner. This, to my knowledge, is the first attempt to put it all together in a personal approach, dealing with the human side of all of us.

As you'll note I've had excellent help from a large number of people. I'm strictly an amatuer at this game, who twice became a guinea pig. I've always written books on management. This is my first book on surgery. As I've told my wife, its probably the longest one-week autobiography on record. Hence, I have relied heavily on the professional and technical guidance of a host of others. Several outstanding people have made direct contributions to sections of the book. Others have checked it for accuracy. Their names are cited in appropriate places. Others, whom I will never know by name—or in some cases by face—gave much, too, but I can only thank them obliquely, by my gratitude and the way I treat my fellow man.

I spent much time revisiting the Cleveland Clinic and interviewing doctors, patients, and friends who have had the operation and have tried to note these contributions in the proper place.

In a way, however, I owe nothing to anybody. I owe it all to myself. I've always been an irascible, up-tight type. My ancestors all had heart problems. Hence, what with the foods that I ate and the drinks that I consumed, I claim full credit for my part in the book. I made it possible.

But I do want to pause here and thank my family for putting up with me, not just during the emotionally trying weeks before and after operation, but always. My daughter, Kathleen, typed the text, and if you could see the rough drafts she worked from, you would appreciate the depth of her understanding and patience. Matthew Fox, Acquisitions Editor at Prentice-Hall, was a great source of help. He has worked with me for several years on other books, and his understanding and professional guidance have always been appreciated. If the book does the job it's intended to, you can thank Matt Fox. Karen Skrable, Production Editor at Prentice-Hall, was of great help for her work in editing the text. She made it readable. In addition to the medical staffs mentioned in the text, Frank Weaver and Ellen Gambrill of the Department of Public Affairs, Cleveland Clinic Foundation, made several helpful suggestions to improve the accuracy and readability of the text. To all these people I am very indebted and very grateful.

INTRODUCTION

WILLIAM P. SHELDON, M.D.
Head of the Department of Cardiology
Cleveland Clinic Foundation

In 1982, some 150,000 coronary artery bypass operations were performed in this country, consuming approximately 2 percent of our total national expenditure for health. A rather remarkable fact considering that only fifteen years have elapsed since this operation was introduced, and as with any new technology, it has experienced its share of controversy. Although the syndrome of angina pectoris and its relationship to coronary sclerosis was recognized in the late 1700s, the clinical recognition of heart attack or acute myocardial infarction did not occur for more than a hundred years, until its description by Herrick in 1912. Nearly fifty years later, in 1958, coronary arteriography provided the opportunity to correlate symptoms with anatomy in the living human. Although open heart surgery became a reality with the development of heart-lung machines a decade earlier, specific attempts to extend the vascular surgical techniques to the coronary artery circulation awaited the development of coronary arteriography—not only to identify suitable candidates but, more important, to measure the value of such operations. After ten years and a myriad of short-lived surgical approaches, the concept of coronary artery bypass grafting seemed, in 1967, to be a major breakthrough: Its beneficial effect upon symptoms was immediate and unequivocal. The advent of an apparently effective surgical alternative challenged scientific methodology for evaluating complex technology and stimulated an explosion of new knowledge regarding the anatomy, physiology, and clinical course of coronary atherosclerosis.

It is not particularly remarkable that this new technology has had a major impact on the practice of cardiovascular medicine and has contributed to escalating health care costs in this country. Among more than 4 million Americans with coronary heart disease, 550,000 die of heart attacks each year. Although coronary artery bypass surgery is still relatively new and is continually being refined and tested, there is agreement that improving blood supply to the heart muscle improves symptoms and restores more normal effort tolerance, and it improves longevity in patients with high-risk types of coronary artery disease. Moreover, preliminary evidence suggests that it may reduce the frequency of hospitalizations and forestalls heart attacks. It does not arrest or cure arteriosclerosis, nor does it reverse the effect that heart attacks have had upon the heart muscle. That must be left to drug treatment and preventive medicine.

Under ideal circumstances, coronary artery bypass surgery can be performed with a mortality risk of 1 percent and a similar risk for complications of heart attack and stroke. These risks become greater if extensive damage to the heart muscle has already occurred or if there is widespread arteriosclerosis involving other organ systems as well. The ultimate objective of the operation is to help the patient achieve life goals through optimal rehabilitation at minimal risk, expense, and inconvenience. Today a seven-day postoperative convalescence in the hospital is commonplace, and most patients are restored to a normal life style in one to two months.

Although prolongation of life is achievable, this results in exposure to other hazards, not the least of which is progression of the arteriosclerotic process. The reality of this observation has led surgeons to become more aggressive in performing primary operations, connecting bypass grafts to less than severely diseased arteries with the hope of preventing repeat operations should the condition progress. Despite this, most centers are experiencing a growing tendency for repeat operations. Nyles Reinfeld is one such patient.

This book describes Reinfeld's personal fight for survival. It is an example of man helping man, or one patient helping others to understand the mysteries of coronary heart disease and its treatment. It is an intimate and deeply personal description of his anxieties, frustrations, and victories, embellished by touches of wry wit. It is a sensitive statement of his personal philosophy and a critical analysis of modern health economics and current hospital systems. Without imparting false optimism or unwarranted pessimism, Reinfeld describes his two-time experience with bypass graft surgery with the intent of providing a perspective for others facing similar decisions. But progress does not end with the final chapter. Results of surgery continue to improve. Nonsurgical alternatives are emerging. Emergency interventions to prevent heart-muscle damage are being explored, and dozens of new medications are helping to improve the medical alternatives. Most important, the patient, through efforts such as Reinfeld's, has become better informed, and the prevention of coronary atherosclerosis, as witnessed by declining mortality figures over the past twenty years, is closer to becoming a reality than ever before.

THE
DEVELOPING PROBLEM

Bewilderment.
The Family Doctor

When you start having heart problems, you don't know whether to be frightened or relieved. Your thoughts focus narrowly on dying and courage. Will I have enough courage?, you wonder.

All our lives we've known that death was a constant companion. Companion, yes, but never a friend, you say! Like Faust and his mischievous associate Mephistopheles, we have enjoyed the precarious pleasures and associations of youth. We have tweaked Old Death's nose more than once and teased him mercilessly, but he always obligingly kept his distance. He was so patient and understanding. He never seemed to be ready to collect—only to threaten from a distance. Suddenly everything is real. He's at the door.

It's like a dream. A bad dream taken out of a movie.

My banker friend and I used to chat on Saturday mornings, when he wasn't too busy, and we'd plan methods for looting the bank. Naturally, we'd be clever enough to not get caught. We considered manipulating the computer, transferring large sums to a secret account in Switzerland. Then we'd slip out of the country, unobserved and unsuspected, and with the money we would set up housekeeping on a Caribbean island. There we'd surround ourselves with beautiful girls, sending checks to our wives to live on. But we never really expected to plunder the bank; at least, I don't think we did. We toyed with it just for fun. Now the cops are banging on the door, in a drama far more real and serious.

Everything has happened so suddenly. So unfairly. There are so many things to be done. So many places to see. So many fences to mend. Why weren't we warned that this would happen? Why weren't we prepared ahead of time?

Of course, I really did have some warning. All kinds of it, in fact. Old Death kept getting closer, but I pretended it was my imagination, or somebody else that looked like him. After

9

all, indigestion and heartburn are caused by gas on the stomach and eating the wrong foods.

When I first saw Death, his nose was just visible above the horizon, like Kilroy. I was just a kid at the time, and he frightened me then, but he kept his distance, and I got over the fear and even taunted him. Next time I saw him, though, his whole head was visible.

It happened at a speech I gave in St. Louis almost ten years ago. I had eaten a big meal at a banquet, accompanied by a few drinks, and got up to speak before a thousand people. I spoke for a minute or two and suddenly came down with an enormous case of indigestion. I stopped talking and just stood still, waiting for it to pass. People looked up at me curiously, to see what was wrong. I said nothing, and it proved to be an excellent attention getter and one of my most dramatic pauses. The pain disappeared as quickly as it came, and I finished the speech. It scared me for a moment or two; the fact that I still remember it indicates that the event registered on my mind, even though I soon forgot or ignored it. I admit that when the pain hit I wondered whether to have my host call an ambulance. Then I was relieved to see the pain pass.

My next view of the Advancing Apparition came one balmy night in Dallas, Texas. His appearance was less startling this time, but it did set me to thinking. But not for long; not long enough to see a doctor. I figured that would be silly.

I was staying at a new hotel on the outskirts of the city. Because I like walking, and because I was on expenses and wanted to keep the cabfare for myself, I decided to walk to the center of town and eat at my favorite restaurant. As I walked it darkened, and I soon found myself in the heart of the most unsavory neighborhood. Street lights became fewer and dimmer, the buildings became more in need of paint and repair, people were standing on the corners, and someone always seemed to be following me. Several times he turned off into some dark doorway, but immediately someone else would come out of the dark and take his place. There were no cabs to catch, so I walked faster. The distance was over five miles, and, as I hurried, my chest began to burn. It felt like an elbow was being pressed against it. As the downtown lights approached and the streets became more friendly, I slowed up and the pain went away. I shrugged it off and ate a hearty meal. I took a cab back to the hotel after having a few drinks.

I next noticed that cold weather began to bother me. Walking the dog on a very cold night, I'd get the same pains. So I quit walking the dog. I let him run loose. It was too cold for anyone to be out then, anyway. At first the dog wouldn't go out alone, because he didn't want out there in the cold either. I'd push him out and duck back into the warm, and pretend not to hear him scratching at the door.

These conditions, which had been infrequent, became more regular and began to be expected. They were not entirely predictable, but they began to affect my way of life, or at least I began to make allowances for them.

My wife and I had always enjoyed eating out late at night. It made the occasion more precious and memorable. When I went to Mexico as a consultant, I ate as late as the Mexicans and enjoyed it. But those times were coming to an end. Heavy eating and a shared bottle of wine now began to keep me awake most of the night. Heartburn and heavy congestion became a problem.

About this time, while serving as chairman of the board of a manufacturing firm with several plants, the president and I flew to Utah to discuss a plant site with the development department. After the meeting, the president and I had dinner in the glass-enclosed restaurant on top of the Hotel Utah in Salt Lake City. The view at night was spectacular. From the restaurant you could look down over the softly lighted Mormon Square with its beautiful temple and historic tabernacle. Snow was falling lightly, and a sense of tranquility permeated the air. After we ate, we walked casually through the square, and then, since the hotel did not serve drinks, we decided to walk to a nearby club. We had two drinks and, since it was late, headed back to the hotel. The distance was only four blocks; it hardly seemed necessary to take a cab. But it was bitter cold outside, and I found myself stopping every few feet to relax the pains in my chest. I was relieved to enter the lobby of the hotel. I had always liked walking, but it was becoming clear that my walking days were limited.

The elbow in my chest was a constant companion by now. I blamed it on an ulcer, because my stomach also seemed to be sensitive to the touch. Maybe it was cancer.

I have since found out that heart attacks and heart problems are as variable as the wind. Some persons have heart attacks and suffer heart damage with no pain; others have extreme pain and suffer no heart damage. The symptoms are also widely varied. Ulcers, for example, get blamed in some cases. In others, people think they're having a gallbladder attack; still others blame it on indigestion and gas. It may even be a backache, shortness of breath, or a numbing sensation in the left arm, which is the most common of all.

One man I met at the Cleveland Clinic, when I was writing this book, had had a complete physical the year before. They found he had an enlarged heart, but no other symptoms. Later he began developing gas pains that ran up his stomach and chest to his neck. Even then the red flag did not go up. The doctor suggested that he keep in touch and that he check back regularly, but he felt the problem was the man's gallbladder. The man, who was a machinist, returned to work. He went back to his doctor the next day in severe pain, and they rushed him to the hospital. He almost didn't survive.

Part of the problem, therefore, is early diagnosis and a patient who keeps his doctor informed.

Since it's easier to avoid the truth than face it, I almost missed the boat.

It was a week or so after my trip to Utah that my son Nick came down with a bad cold. I took him to our family doctor (really two doctors, who work as a team: Drs. James F. Grow, Jr., and William E. Moats, both very able and dedicated men). Quite by chance, the doctor asked me how I was doing, and I mentioned the pain in my chest and the symptoms. He gave me a cardiogram on the spot and sent me immediately to the hospital for tests, in our local paramedic ambulance.

The tests showed that three of the arteries leading to the heart were badly occluded. Dr. A.P. Ormond, Jr., the cardiologist who performed the heart catheterization, advised me of the findings and made the recommendation that I have bypass surgery. By now I'd had enough pain and discomfort that the solution he proposed was not entirely unexpected or unwanted. Besides, I was curious enough as an individual to be interested in the experience, even in being one of the first. On the other hand, the idea wasn't so appealing when considered from the standpoint that it was my life that was on the line.

I asked him where he suggested getting it done. He advised me that the operation could be done right in Akron, or I could have my choice. By now I had begun to like him and to trust him, so I asked to meet the surgeon. The next day my wife Ginny and I met him, a youthful man named Dr. John Hansel. Besides being young, he was also small and short, so he looked like a high school kid who'd been working afternoons as a busboy in the hospital kitchen. Hardly the type to inspire confidence. He had the long, slender fingers of a surgeon, however, and besides, as my wife pointed out later, he was extremely good looking; so, having passed the two most important tests, we both voted to have Dr. Hansel do the honors. But as a final act of reassurance, I asked Dr. Hansel what his batting average was. He looked me over carefully, as if checking my own qualifications, and then told me I would be his thirty-third open heart patient. My face must have lighted up and then clouded over. He sensed that I was wondering how many of those thirty-two had survived but was afraid to ask. So he answered for me: "All of them."

With odds like these in my favor, how could I turn down the chance to be number thirty-three? Even the Cleveland Clinic or another famous hospital in the nation couldn't compete against this record. So I said, "Go ahead," thinking for the moment almost as if it were my wife who was going to be operated on instead of me. But when he left, reality struck and I wanted to call him back and think about it. I had in fact earlier asked Dr. Ormond if I could wait—indefinitely. Unfortunately, my condition posed a serious immediate threat, and waiting might be fatal. But then, the operation could be, too, I thought to myself. And the operation was scheduled for two days hence, and my natural demise might be months away. Maybe the thing to do was to time the two events closer together like Constantine and his baptism. My wife once again broke my chain of thought by mentioning how handsome Dr. Hansel was; so, after weighing all the facts on the scale, in the best traditions of management I accepted my wife's wiser judgment and had the operation—never dreaming for a moment that there might be some form of sinister plot involved here.

Since I wouldn't be writing this if I had died, you know that Dr. Hansel did a most creditable job. I survived and so did his conscience—and he couldn't blame me for ruining a perfect record.

There's more to come, thanks to this skillful knife wielder. Actually much more, because it was almost exactly six years later that I came back for another operation.

It wasn't that I enjoyed the first one that much. It was, in fact, rather unpleasant. And I had no desire to see either of the doctors again, nor to test Dr. Hansel's batting average. They were great guys, but there are limits to this sort of thing. No; unfortunately my problem was poor plumbing—a defect that began with the original design. Like an old house with rusty plumbing, replacing a section here and there was no substitute for the ravages of time. In fact, they couldn't even use new material like a plumber would. Because the body rejects foreign material, they borrowed plumbing out of the basement to replace the restricted areas around my heart. They stripped a vein out of my leg and spliced it into my heart in two places. After five years or so, this reluctant transplant sealed itself up, and I was back in trouble. So it was back to the drawing board.

From what I understand now, five to six years is about the cycle for those first patients of bypass surgery who return for seconds. Newer knowledge and better technology are extending this cycle, so that patients undergoing the operation today can probably hope for many more years before they come back again. They may even outlive their doctors, and wreak their final revenge.

My second operation was exactly one week before Christmas; my new set of symptoms had begun to be a problem in the spring.

I coached a soccer team in the spring, made up of young teenagers. When we began practice in April, the weather was often cold and rainy. We even had some snow. And yet I worked with the kids in that cold, damp weather without too many problems. My main symptoms were a tightening of the jaw and throat along with a dull pain. At its worst, it was difficult to speak because my jaw was very stiff.

My chest would also get to burning inside when I was too active. The only position I could play was goalie, which I did on occasion when we split the group into two teams at the end of each practice session. I don't know if those kids even knew about my problem. They probably figured I was just a lazy coach. Most amateur coaches seem to have beer bellies. They don't look very athletic. They stand and shout instructions to the kids, like a drill sergeant. The kids eat it up and never question the old principle; "Do as I say, not as I do." As a result, it was easy for me to cheat. Besides, my son Nick was on the team, and he probably covered up for me.

When I ran, I loped. But the kids charged full tilt across the field. If I ran a hundred feet, I stopped and rested my hands on my knees and panted for breath. The kids ran for miles. The kids probably laughed at my faltering gait behind my back, but they were too polite to let me know. We had fun, though, and they did a terrific job.

My career as a coach had begun a month earlier, when I decided to take a class run by three soccer coaches from the University of Akron. There were about sixty of us fathers and several mothers in attendance. I signed up for the course because I thought it would be in a classroom where I could sit down and listen. I was mistaken. To make matters worse, I was the oldest man in the group. I was in my fifties. The others ranged from their twenties to thirties; maybe an occasional forty. Furthermore, none of them had potbellies. They all looked like varsity athletes just out of high school. The name of the game was learning by doing. First there was a lecture, then a do-it-yourself session on the gym floor. Exercises. Running games. Endurance tests. Challenges of one-on-one and many-against-many. Every few minutes, the coach would pick someone from the crowd to challenge him on a point or to work him until he nearly dropped, to prove how durable the body was. Every time the coach began his search for a volunteer, I ducked out of sight behind someone. I learned to keep out of sight and as far to the rear as I could. When the whole group was on the floor playing strenuous games, I would sneak out the door of the gym and pretend to make a phone call. I had more important calls to make during that course than if I'd been back in the office.

I only got caught once. The coach needed a volunteer, and I was conspicuously visible behind my shield. Coaches really aren't as dumb as I thought. He knew I was avoiding him. And he may have sensed why. At any rate, he took it easy on me, and we both saved face. The course lasted for two weekends, all day long. It was followed by a written exam, and believe it or not, I passed and am now a certified soccer coach.

I confess I had a lot of doubts about my sanity during that course. What was I doing in a high-physical-activity sport? I was embarrassed because of my age and because of my handicap.

During the preceding five years, following the operation, I had been more active physically than at any time since I got married. But this spring I noticed a marked slowing down, more angina and more discomfort with less freedom of move-ment. My physical energy wasn't there like it had been. I had to push myself more. My chest pained me and burnt more.

During the first five years, I doubt if I took five nitro-glycerin tablets in the whole time. I was now taking maybe three or four a week.

Sometimes while coaching a soccer game I had trouble. Other times there were no visible signs of angina, even in cool weather.

I'd had a number of strange pains over the past few years. A sudden stabbing pain that seemed to move across the chest and then disappear as quickly as it came. Sharp tingling in my left arm with a dull ache at the top. Pains in the top of my shoulders like someone was pinching me hard. Sometimes these would last a few minutes, sometimes for days. Pains up the back of my neck, in my throat, in my stomach. How do you know what these pains are? When the doctor would ask, on my periodic visit, if I was having any pains, what could I answer? Some pains were so old they had become a part of my life and I had come to accept them. Frequently, I didn't know what to tell the doctor. Sometimes I hated to sound like a complainer asking for sympathy. Sometimes it was easier to shrug it off because the pain was gone at the time I talked to him. Have you ever noticed how your aches and pains seem to disappear just when you see the doctor? You could have been vomiting every ten minutes with the flu that day, but as soon as he enters the examination room, you're feeling better, and you start wondering why you're there. Sometimes there isn't time to talk to him.

My wife once accused me of telling more to the nurse than I did to the doctor, and I think this is true. My daughter Carol, who's a registered nurse, also confirms that this happens to her. Men don't like to reveal themselves to other men. They find it easier to talk to women. Maybe it's because of the mother complex or male ego. Perhaps all male doctors should have male patients interviewed by a female nurse ahead of time. Then the doctor can read her notes and find out what's going on. Instead, the doctor suddenly appears in the examination room; his lobby is jammed with people, and he has several patients in various states of undress in other rooms. He is obviously eager to finish before midnight, so he marches up to you and attempts to combine conversation with physical analysis. "Hello, how are you doing?" he asks. Then, while you make the mistake of answering with pleasantries, before launching into your rehearsed list of complaints, he puts his stethoscope on your back and says, "Breathe deeply through your mouth." (Or if he's a dentist, he waits till your mouth is full before he starts asking questions. "Just nod your head," he says cheerfully, as he carries on his canned monologue.) He checks your blood pressure. Again you feel duty-bound to keep quiet so as not to affect the reading. Then he says, "Keep taking the medication." As he leaves the room, he says, "You can put your shirt back on. I'm glad to see you're doing so well. See you in four months," and he's gone—off to see the next bewildered patient.

Following my first operation, I had made a practice of either walking or riding a bike for about an hour each day. In the winter, I was one of the "walkers" at the mall. In the summer, I walked the neighborhood. I was a street walker. Thus it happened that one summer night, following my coaching career, my wife and I set out to walk around the block. Usually I walk faster than she, and it is I who has to slow down, but this time she kept getting ahead of me. I had trouble getting back home. Half way, I had to stop and allow the angina to subside. A year earlier, I could have walked that block ten times without incident. My problems were mounting. My condition had worsened.

These problems were reemphasized later on a trip to Washington, D.C., in the fall. The weather was cool and damp. For convenience, I stayed at the Hyatt near the subway station. The walk of only one block to the subway became very difficult. Every walk in the city was a problem. I wasn't short of breath. It was the angina again. The same old enemy: the burning and tension in my chest and jaw. It was worse after meals. When I left the hotel, I began skipping breakfast to make it easier to get through the morning.

By late fall and early winter, angina was keeping me awake at night, sometimes until early morning. I began to get angina watching TV after dinner. By now I was taking as many as five or six nitroglycerin tablets per day. I could no longer walk at the mall with the old vigor. I used to make six round trips an hour; now I struggled to make two.

My chest always felt congested, like it had a belt around it or as if I had been pumped up like an inflated ball. At times my stomach stuck out from the air I had gulped. I burped a lot, constantly trying to relieve the pressure. (It used to work when I had indigestion.) I'd wake up in the middle of the night and would go to the bathroom, searching for anything to deflate the balloon inside me. A hot shower, steaming hot, on my back seemed to help the most. When the heat sank in, I would start burping, feeling better for a few minutes. The heat probably helped my circulation. One of my friends at the mall joined me one day. As we walked, he complained that his angina was bothering him. He mentioned, purely by chance, that burping always helped him when he was having problems.

Sensing the seriousness of my own situation, I called my insurance agent and asked him to increase my coverage. Fortune smiled and my timing was excellent. The extra coverage was granted. (The company knew of my medical history.)

I also made notes of detailed instructions for cleaning up

my affairs and went over them with my wife, so she wouldn't have to pick up the stray ends unprepared.

Then, the morning before Thanksgiving, two weeks after my return from Washington, I awoke at 3 A.M. with a tremendous chest pain. I was soaked with perspiration. I slipped nitro tablets under my tongue, but they gave little relief. I sat on the edge of the bed for a while, then woke my wife. Gradually the pain subsided, but not completely. Thanksgiving Day I hardly ate anything. Our married children and their families came over for dinner, but I didn't feel good enough to enjoy their company. I felt weak, like I had the flu; I was sick to my stomach and generally unfit. Over the past few years, colds had bothered me a great deal, causing breathing problems. So even now I hated to admit my problem was as severe as it was. I hoped it was the result of the flu, but deep down I knew the truth. That old Apparition had finally gotten through the front door.

I worked the Friday after Thanksgiving, going to several business meetings. About 3 P.M., I went up to the mall and walked, but it was very unpleasant. A friend joined me for a few minutes, but it was difficult for me to keep up, even though he was in his seventies. At my wife's urging, I finally went to see our family doctor, the team of Moats and Grow. Drs. Moats and Grow are unique among their profession. They are compassionate as well as thorough. They leave little to chance and aren't inclined to hand you an aspirin and tell you everything will be all right. I know this from experiences with my children. That in itself is reassuring, but it's also the moment of truth. It wasn't an easy decision to see the doctor, because I knew what he would do.

I guess I had been hoping that if I kept going long enough, it would all eventually pass like a nightmare, and everything would be OK. That's how it was when I was younger. But now, by going to the doctor, I was admitting that I no longer controlled my fate. It was almost like giving up, and when that happens there isn't much hope.

The doctor ran a cardiogram and ordered me to the hospital at once. He wanted to call an ambulance, but I insisted that I had been driving about all day and that I could drive myself. He was very hesitant. It was most unusual, he said, to have a patient drive to the hospital and then be admitted to intensive care. But I could only see myself scaring the family badly if I went in an ambulance. I remember the first ambulance ride, six years earlier, when my boy was only nine. He seemed to be so frightened and worried. I would never want to inflict that sadness on anyone again. I promised to go straight home, pack, and let my wife drive me to the hospital, which I did. It was a long, sad ride that evening.

In the meantime, the doctor called ahead and arranged to have me admitted to intensive care. I was once more removed from the warmth and security of my family. My future looked grim indeed.

Obviously, as we all know but too infrequently admit, the patient who has himself for a doctor has a fool for a doctor.

It wouldn't be fair for me to leave this chapter in midair without a more serious discussion of the problem. In my own view, I saw the problem subjectively, as you have seen. I saw it as the victim, emotionally and personally. I was little interested in the fineness of detail and the expert finesse of the trained practitioner.

In this respect the problems discussed and my reactions were probably similar to those that others have felt. Your own life and survival, however, may depend upon a much more sober response and understanding of the problem, and this requires the professional hand, as will be explained by Dr. Moats.

You may wonder, at times, why doctors themselves don't do a better job of analyzing the problems. I have done this myself at times, and then I get to thinking of the tremendously complex organism that the body is—of the many similar and conflicting symptoms that the body signals to tell us it's in need of help. Different illnesses, for example, can send out the same signals. These have to be analyzed, weighed, and evaluated. One by one the search must be made, discarding possibilities and testing new ones. We take our car to the garage and complain that the garages never fix the problem. I often say that you have to take your car in twice to get the simplest things fixed. Garages never seem to get it right the first time.

Doctors don't have this luxury, and they are dealing with

a much more complex system. Furthermore, you probably do a better job of describing your car's symptoms than you do in describing your own. When you talk about yourself, you tend to become subjective and to skip over things that embarrass you or seem insignificant. With your car, on the other hand, the first few months you own it, you note down every strange squeek and rattle, giving a long list to the garage mechanic to guide him. No such care and detail usually attends the patient's contact with a doctor.

Quite the contrary. As patients, we unconsciously make the doctor's job harder in the very area that is most important to us. We challenge the doctor to save our life, as if it were a test of will. But don't take my word for it. Read what Dr. Moats, one of my favorite doctors, has to say. Dr. Moats, by the way, is the type of professionally dedicated individual that we all hope to find as our family doctor. He once considered going into professional baseball, and it is baseball's loss and humanity's good fortune that he did not. He is still active in sports and serves as the team doctor for my son's football team. He has a very busy schedule; the fact that he took the time to write this in the middle of his busiest season is an indication of his concern. It is also a source of great personal satisfaction to me.

THE SAME PROBLEM FROM A PROFESSIONAL POINT OF VIEW
William E. Moats, M.D.
Diplomate American Board of Family Practice

The frantic phone call by a patient's spouse alerting the family physician to an in-progress heart attack can produce a very difficult and traumatic experience. As a family physician, I have far too often encountered this type of call from a spouse imploring me to respond quickly to his or her mate's massive myocardial infarction. Unfortunately, any response may well come too late.

Over the last several years, great strides have been made in the care of the acute heart attack patient. For example, the medical profession has undertaken a far-reaching educational program for prehospital coronary care by developing highly trained and skilled paramedics who are qualified to initiate and sustain cardiopulmonary function until the emergency ward is reached. Because time is a critical factor in heart emergencies, every moment saved is extremely important in the management of the acute heart patient. Many times the delay in transportation from the emergency room to the coronary care unit (CCU) can be eliminated by transporting the patient directly to the coronary care unit by the emergency medical team. Once in the CCU, the ultrasophisticated equipment and techniques and, most important, the highly skilled medical staff take over, assuring the patient of the utmost in care to help him or her survive a major injury to the heart.

All that I have alluded to deals with time: the speedy response of the emergency squad, the rapid transportation to the hospital CCU, and the immediate care by the personnel there. This is great and it works. But wait a minute. Let's stop patting our collective medical backs. Haven't we forgotten several very important steps? What have we done to impress on our patients their responsibility in completing the cycle? Have we convinced them to call for help immediately when symptoms occur instead of waiting an hour or two before seeking medical assistance? (By then it could be too late.) Have we, as family physicians, impressed enough upon the patient the risk factors of coronary heart disease? Have we encouraged our patients to enroll in a cardiopulmonary resuscitation (CPR) course so that they can be as knowledgeable as possible in carrying out CPR? (What a hopeless feeling for the family doctor to be on the wrong end of the telephone when a wife calls and is unable to assist her unconscious husband because she doesn't know how. CPR can't be taught over the phone in an emergency situation.) Have we also made the general public aware of the signs and symptoms of an acute heart attack? Patient education and response are perhaps the most important aspect of the cycle, without which the skilled care may be totally wasted.

What can the family doctor do about this? He can make speeches at civic meetings, such as Rotary, Kiwanis, church groups, and so on, to help get the message across. Better yet, he can meet with the patient in a one-on-one encounter to define the risk of developing arteriosclerotic heart disease (ASHD). An initial examination, perhaps a complete physical examination, enables the physician to uncover any of the risk factors and symptoms of ASHD in the patient.

What are the risk factors of coronary artery disease? Simply stated, they are as follows:

1. Family history of heart disease
2. Hypertension
3. Obesity
4. Smoking
5. High cholesterol levels in the blood

Any one or combination of these is sufficient to alert the family physician to potential problems. Becoming acquainted with the patient also helps. Is he a Type A (high-strung, nervous) individual or a Type B (laid-back, easygoing) person?

The signs and symptoms of a heart attack are many, and the variants are beyond the scope of this presentation. The classical description of a myocardial infarction will suffice. The patient has the onset of a heavy, oppressive, widespread, viselike, squeezing pain in his chest that is difficult to localize and not necessarily related to exertion. It may radiate to the neck, jaw, arms, or abdomen. The pain may be accompanied by nausea and vomiting, profuse diaphoresis (sweating), and a feeling of impending doom. Most patients do not feel like moving around to relieve the pain. If the patient experiences a sharp, well-localized chest pain made worse by motion, breathing, coughing, or sneezing, this is not likely to be cardiac in origin. But any chest pain should be thoroughly evaluated. As a family physician, I'd rather my patients be wrong several times and have it evaluated than be right once and not pursue it. "Being a live coward is better than being a dead hero."

Most patients have prior warning of a potential heart attack. That statement might be taken to task by some cardiologists, but I believe it is true. Undue shortness of breath on exertion, a toothache or shoulder discomfort when walking in a cold wind, mild chest pain on exertion, all may signify an approaching heart attack. The recognition and follow-up of some of these vague symptoms would perhaps ensure that more of our patients would benefit from the banks of medical technology.

As a family physician, I am usually made aware of a potential heart problem in one of three ways: (1) The asymptomatic individual comes to me for evaluation of the aforementioned risk factors. Appropriate studies are obtained (cholesterol, triglycerides, high-density lipoprotein, serum profile, stress ECG), and cardiology consultation is obtained if indicated. (2) A symptomatic patient presents me with one or more of the warning symptoms of coronary insufficiency (angina pectoris), and more rapid evaluation and treatment are undertaken. (3) By far the least desirable is the sometimes catastrophic presentation of an acute myocardial infarction and all its potential complications.

Heart patients respond to their illness in so many different ways, from the extremely frightened and apprehensive to the denying stoic (who is probably also very frightened). My response to the patient's illness can certainly become entangled in a web of emotions, particularly if the patient and his or her family is quite close to me professionally or socially. My primary goal, no matter what my emotions, is to obtain for that patient the ultimate in care as quickly and efficiently as I can. Assuming his or her proper role, the family physician becomes a coordinator of medical care, liaison, counselor, and friend to the patient and family during the hospital stay and treatment. More often than not, the family will call the family physician, rather than the cardiologist, concerning the patient's status. This seems appropriate, for it is the family physician who will provide the long-term support for the patient and family after the hospital stay.

3

TESTS,
HEART CATHETERIZATION,
AND INTENSIVE CARE

*Frustration
and Anger*

When you leave the security of your family doctor, he transfers you to the hands of a specialist. You now enter the strange world of the hospital and meet only strangers. The walls and floor are cold tile, and you end up in a peculiar gown that's split up the back; you loose all your clothes, which are sent home. You keep your watch.

What a disgusting, disturbing experience! Everything that was ever familiar and comfortable is gone.

They stick foam rubber pads to your chest and hook wires to them. Over your head is a heart monitor that shows your cardiogram on a TV scope. For entertainment you watch the scope and see the blips indicating each heartbeat. You study the pattern of the cardiogram. It doesn't look the way it did when you were younger, getting an annual physical. At that time, there was a blip, then a flat line, then another blip, and so on. Now the graph has a curved shape and extra spikes. In another place on the machine, an LCD counter shows the heartbeat in beats per minute. If you keep very still, you can watch your pulse slow down and then speed up as you move. These signals also are transmitted to a central nurse's station, where a nurse looks up to check you, if the signals send her an alarm.

You go to the toilet in a bedpan. As any patient in a hospital knows, this is the signal for the nurse to come in, or for visitors to arrive without warning. Have you ever tried to go in a bedpan with visitors in the room?

For medication, they tape a yellowish salve to your skin. This is a long-acting, continuous-action nitroglycerin that is used in place of pills placed under the tongue. This was a new development. Instead of taking medicine orally, say every four hours, you pasted it on your skin and absorbed it into the blood for four hours.

Taken this way, nitroglycerin gives you a terrific headache. There is no cure, apparently, for any ill that doesn't at times make the illness itself seem like an improvement!

Somewhere along the line, you get to feeling better and you wonder why you're there. Maybe you sold the doctor a bill of goods and things aren't as serious as they seemed.

By the next morning, you are ready to go home, but they have other ideas.

Blood tests are taken every few hours. Dracula could not find a better place to make his home.

It seems that every ten minutes a nurse is in your room doing something to you. Checking your pulse. Checking your blood pressure. Taking your temperature. Getting specimens. Measuring the amount you void. Seeing if you're all right.

Every intern in the hospital stops by to practice his trade. Everyone, it seems, wants your life history. It starts the night you check in, and you wonder why they don't compare notes and save time.

Finally your family doctor arrives, and your whole morning lights up at the sight of a familiar face. But he does little more than say hello and wish you well. Then he's off to light some other patient's life. You are now in the hands of the cardiologist.

My cardiologist was Dr. Ormond, the man who had shepherded me through the first operation. He had kept tabs on me at regular intervals during the intervening period, so he was called in by Dr. Moats and Dr. Grow when I entered the hospital.

Dr. Ormond visited briefly, but his comments were noncommittal, other than to advise me of the need to run more tests.

Later that day I was moved to another room and put on a kind of "beeper system." A portable transmitter was hooked up to my chest, and the signal was sent by radio to the nurse's station. I was allowed, now, to go to the bathroom, but I had to call a nurse to assist me in getting out of bed. I had suddenly become an invalid. Once I forgot and got up by myself, and a drill sergeant, in the guise of a nurse, informed me that that was forbidden.

Her sudden appearance without warning reminded me of the story they tell in the shop: The only time you can find the boss is when you make a mistake. That's when he walks in, just in time to catch you.

The call button on the pillow next to your head is a useless luxury serving the same purpose in reverse. When you check in, they tell you to press the button when you need the nurse, and she'll be right in. But you need the patience of Job to make it work. The nurse never hears it. The best way to get her attention is to detach a couple of the wires from your chest. This sends her the signal that you're dead, and she comes rushing in. Even here you must be prudent, because you're only allowed to die so many times accidentally before she becomes suspicious. I don't know what would happen after that, if you really did die. She'd probably rehook you up to the wires and go on about her work.

An even more exciting prospect is to visualize the poor, overworked nurse, who faces a whole ward of patients, who all disconnect at once. Such are the joys and excitement of life in a hospital room. There's nothing like it on the outside. It's times like these that try a man's soul and a nurse's patience.

Next morning I was visited by Dr. Ormond, who advised me that he felt I should have a heart catheterization. I nodded my head glumly. The catheterization was scheduled for the next morning.

This was to be my third time for this procedure. The first catheterization preceded my first operation; the second was several months later, to check the results of the operation.

That evening a representative from Dr. Ormond's office came to my room to instruct me on the procedure for the catheterization. She was a pretty young nurse named Linda Insalago, who smiled easily at my morbid sense of humor. This was fortunate for me, because I had spent most of my free time in the afternoon entertaining myself by making notes on the tawdry condition of my room, and I needed someone to relate my findings to. She was perfect, because she seemed to understand and agree, at least to my face. Her pleasantness oiled my tongue, and I'm afraid I took advantage of her.

I might not have noticed this room myself under normal circumstances. Being a management consultant, I travel considerably and stay in hotels and motels of all sorts. As a result, I have become unduly critical of my surroundings and habitat.

Hence, I noticed the room and it took little to upset me. The overhead lamp was broken. The paint on the walls was scratched. The paint around the wooden window frame was blistered and cracked. The drapes and shades were darkened by loose dirt, and both were torn. The chair and dresser were badly beaten up from years of scuffing about. The radiator was blackened with soot of long standing. Soot and dust were in the cracks and corners of the floor tile. "How is it possible to relate these conditions to the public image of sanitary cleanliness and sterility?" I asked poor Mrs. Insalago. "Aren't dirt and filth the scourge of the hospital? Of the sick?" I went on, looking to her for an answer. What could she say? I had her cornered.

"Many of these conditions are the result of years of accumulation," I continued. She edged toward the door, but I moved to block her exit. "A scratch on a new paint job is to be expected in a hospital, or even in a well-kept hotel. But maintenance and attention to detail are also expected. Why, one time when I was visiting a major steel company," I interjected importantly, "my associate and I walked through the plant to look over the operation. As we walked, my friend kicked at the material blocking our way and said sharply, 'Housekeeping is a sign of the quality of management. There is a direct correlation.'

"And so it is for all types of businesses," I added on my own. Mrs. Insalago looked at me sympathetically, as if she realized that this might be my last important speech. She had almost made it to the doorway, edging around me.

"This hospital, for all its excellent doctors and fine nurses—which I really believe to be true—shows clear signs of poor administration and inattention to human needs and desires," I said, grabbing her arm and holding her from leaving.

"As you would guess, the food is equally bad. Everyone apologizes for hospital food: 'It is bland because it is dietary' or 'They have so many people to serve,'" I said, mimicking those who didn't understand the situation. "But these are excuses for ineptitude and lack of attention. Large restaurants could not survive on these platitudes. The cafeteria that serves the doctors and the visitors is just as bad. My family tried it once and never returned," I shouted at her triumphantly. But Mrs. Insalago had escaped, and with her went my only witness. And I wasn't finished. I wanted to tell her more. I wanted to tell her about the human being inside of me and that I didn't like being there. That I wanted to go home.

As it was I had belabored poor Mrs. Insalago too long about this, and what with the events of the next few weeks, I completely forgot about it. But several months later, in Dr. Ormond's office she asked me, quite to my surprise, if I had mentioned these things to the hospital. I had not. At the time, I felt better for it all, and when Mrs. Insalago completed her instructions to me for the morning, I was ready to tackle the catheter caper next morning and the hospital on my release, but other things interfered—namely, open heart surgery.

Heart catheterization is a specialized diagnostic procedure that consists of slowly passing a very thin, flexible, hollow tube through the vessels of the arm or groin into the chambers of the heart. The tube, or catheter, follows the course of the blood vessels.

The procedure enables the doctor to determine the nature of the heart problem in ways not possible otherwise. As you know, the function of the heart is to pump blood to the billions of cells in the body.

The heart has four chambers, two on each side of a separating wall. On each side of this wall is an upper receiving chamber (atrium) and a lower pumping chamber (ventricle). It is these pumps that circulate the blood.

At the inlet and outlet of each pumping chamber there is a valve, like a trapdoor. These valves keep the blood moving in the proper direction through the heart. All the chambers have muscular walls that contract rhythmically, but the walls of the pumping chambers are the thickest and strongest.

The blood, which has carried oxygen and nourishment to all parts of the body, picks up wastes, such as carbon dioxide, and is then circulated back to the right upper heart chamber (atrium) through two large veins (the IVC and SVC in Fig. 3.1). When the ventricles relax, the accumulated blood causes the inlet valve (1) to open, letting the blood pass from this upper chamber (RA) to the one below (RV). The exit valve (2) at the outlet holds shut while the chamber fills. Then, with

SVC superior vena cava
IVC inferior vena cava
RA right atrium
RV right ventricle
MPA main pulmonary artery
RPA right pulmonary artery
LPA left pulmonary artery
PV pulmonary veins
LA left atrium
LV left ventricle
AORTA

VALVES
1 tricuspid
2 pulmonary
3 mitral
4 aortic

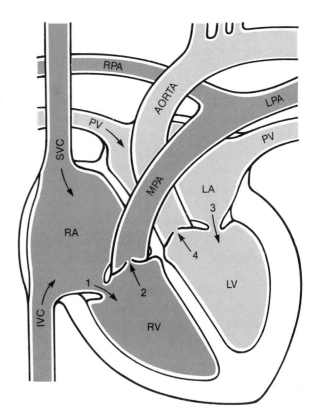

FIGURE 3.1 *(Used by Permission from Chicago Heart Association.)*

a strong contraction, the right ventricle closes its inlet valve (1), opens its outlet valve (2), and pushes its blood into the big pulmonary artery (MPA), whose two main branches carry blood to the lungs. Here, through capillary vessels, the carbon dioxide in the blood is thrown off into the air sacs to go out with the breath, and oxygen is taken in. In this way the blood is changed from purple or dark red (venous) to bright red (arterial).

After leaving the lungs, the blood returns to the upper left chamber of the heart (LA). The left ventricle fills through the valve (3). The left ventricle is the thickest and strongest of all the heart chambers. When it contracts and pushes blood through the exit valve (4), the blood is given a vigorous start into the aorta, the body's largest artery. From here it makes its long trip through the body, in some places running uphill—to the brain, for example—before it returns to the right atrium.

The two coronary arteries, which branch off from the aorta, wind around the heart and supply the heart muscle with oxygen and food (see Fig. 3.2).

A common inborn defect is a hole in the wall separating the two sides of the heart. When this occurs, the blood passes into the wrong places. Blood that has been oxygenated may circulate back to the lungs instead of passing through the arteries. Some blood may not get to the lungs at all but instead circulates through the body still dark for lack of oxygen. This happens to blue babies. In either case, the heart is working inefficiently, and there may not be enough oxygen-carrying blood to fuel the body properly.

Another defect occurs when a heart valve is misshapen or stiffened. This can result from a birth defect or be caused by a disease such as rheumatic fever. In either case, the malfunctioning valve affects the flow of blood, and the heart is forced to work harder. Even then, the flow of blood may not be capable of properly sustaining the body.

In adult life, atherosclerosis, or "hardening of the arteries," may narrow the coronary arteries that supply oxygen and food to the heart muscles. This will not be noticed for a while, but when the arteries become precariously narrow, symptoms develop, such as chest discomfort on exertion, called angina pectoris. These pains warn us that the heart muscle is not getting enough food and oxygen to meet its needs. The heart is sending out warning signals.

Heart catheterization is useful in diagnosing all of these heart problems. Before a catheterization is done, however, a number of simpler studies are made of the heart function. These include learning the nature and history of your symptoms, listening to heart sounds and murmurs with a stethoscope, studying chest x-rays, and obtaining an electrocardiogram of the heart. If these tests indicate that you have one of the types of heart trouble just discussed, the physician then may want a heart catheterization to confirm his diagnosis.

THE CORONARY ARTERIES OF THE HEART

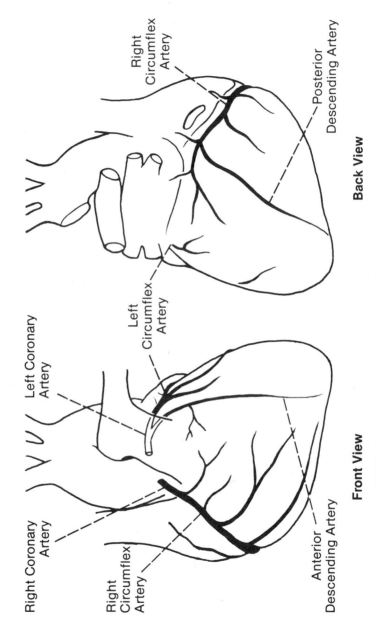

Front View

Back View

FIGURE 3.2 *(Used by Permission from Chicago Heart Association.)*

34

Heart catheterization is the only way in which the doctor can find out with accuracy the severity of the defects in your heart and exactly where they are located. From the information thus gathered, plus other facts he has obtained, he is then able to advise you about the type of surgery or care that will be most helpful in treating your particular condition. It's possible that a major operation may not be necessary. In the six years since my first heart operation a number of advances have been made in dealing with heart problems; this provides much hope for the future. One advance, for example, uses a special catheter to open up the restricted nodule in the artery. This is done by means of a balloon attached to the end of the catheter. When the catheter is inserted in the blood vessel, the balloon is positioned at the location of the restriction. The balloon is then inflated, expanding it against the wall of the artery, forcing the area open, like a plumber's auger. The method is relatively new and not always effective.

I met a man who had had such an operation during my second stay in the hospital. Following my own catheterization, I was wandering along the halls and fell into conversation with an elderly gentleman, who was cheerful despite his problems. As he described his experiences, the balloon technique had been relatively successful at first. It actually had reduced his symptoms, and he was aware of improvement. Unfortunately, the solids which had built up inside the heart artery had reclaimed the area, and in three weeks he was back in the hospital, with the original symptoms or problem. This was when I met him.

Rumors of other techniques mention possible medicines that will work like a plumber's lye to clean out the pipes. But I can see many problems here before a safe method is possible. I would not want to be an early volunteer. As Ponce de León discovered, there is no simple source of eternal youth.

On the day before your heart catheterization, the doctor who will perform the diagnosis will probably examine you. He will want to know the history of your illness, whether you are allergic to anything, whether you have a tendency to abnormal bleeding, or if you are taking medication that will slow coagulation of the blood. This is the time for you to ask questions.

Because I find that I forget the questions I had planned to ask, I have learned to jot them down, like a checklist, to use when I talk to the doctor.

The doctor may ask you to sign a form saying you consent to the test. If the large vessels of the groin are to be used for introduction of the catheter, that area will be shaved. Just before the catheterization you may be given a sedative to help you relax. The actual test takes about one hour, rarely more than two.

During the test, you will be awake. You are strapped to a table to keep you from rolling off, as the table will be rotated left and right in order to place you on one side or the other as needed during the analysis. The table is surrounded by large x-ray apparatus and other equipment, which picks up and records information about your condition. You are also connected to an electrocardiograph so that your heart rate and rhythm can be monitored continuously.

The progress of the catheter is watched on an x-ray TV (see Fig. 3.3) tube, so if you want to, you can watch along with the doctor. This is obviously a learning process for the patient as well as the doctor. Having been through it three times, I feel like an expert. I mentioned to Dr. Ormond that I should now be qualified to start my own practice, with him as my first victim, but he only smiled. He never volunteered. Actually, my offer—which, incidentally, would have cost him nothing (I would have done it free)—was not without its real-life parallel: The man who worked out the procedure in 1929, a German physician named Werner Forsmann, performed the first heart catheterization on himself. I never wanted to go quite that far, however.

During the catheterization procedure, pressures in each heart chamber are measured, blood samples from each part of the heart can be withdrawn for testing, and x-ray contrast material can be inspected through the catheter. All this while, a film of the heart is made with the x-ray apparatus. This is called angiocardiography. It outlines the interior of the heart to show the size of the heart chambers. It also permits any abnormal conditions or leaking heart valves to be seen and measured. If necessary, x-ray contrast material can be introduced into each coronary artery to show any blockage or narrowing. This is called a coronary angiograph.

Heart catheterization imposes a small risk, which depends upon the individual. Only your physician can explain the risk in detail. But the fact that the procedure is often done in newborn babies, and that Dr. Forsmann performed it on himself, indicates how small the risk actually is.

Just before the catheterization you will be given a local anesthetic in the area, arm or groin, where the catheter is going to be introduced, either through a needle or through a small cut in the skin. Often both places are used. Since the area is anesthetized, you do not feel the catheter going in. You may feel it working its way up your arm. Some people feel it in a vague sort of way, and some don't feel it at all. I couldn't feel it in my arm, but I felt a tingling, almost like a slight prickling itch, in my heart as it entered my chest. By and large the procedure is painless. Your heart may skip a beat as the catheter is passed through it. This is normal and expected. The first time it startles you, and you take a quick breath involuntarily.

There is one stage that may be momentarily uncomfortable. This is when the dye is injected into the bloodstream so the heart's action can be seen on x-ray and recorded. For these few seconds there is a burning sensation throughout the body and a bitter taste in the mouth. Some people get a headache or a feeling of nausea. The first time, I got sick to my stomach, and the doctor waited for a few moments until that passed. The last time, perhaps because I was more relaxed and less fearful, I did not become nauseous. In any case, these unpleasant sensations are short-lived, passing quickly. Almost everyone has them, so they should not be unexpected or cause for concern. You will be told when it is going to happen. At times during the test you may be asked to exercise, take deep breaths, or cough.

After the tests are completed, the catheter is withdrawn, and the opening entry points are closed and stitched together. During this final phase, the area is still numb from the anesthesia, so there is no pain or discomfort. Removing the stitches in five or six days is relatively painless, causing a slight twitch like a hair being plucked.

Most doctors hold the patient overnight in the hospital for observation in case delayed symptoms appear after the catheterization. Reactions that may occur are feelings of weak-

FIGURE 3.3 Chest X-Rays Showing Catheters in Place (white line); (a) Here the Catheter Has Passed through the Right Arm Vein, into the Left Pulmonary Artery; (b) Showing Catheter in Main Pulmonary Artery.

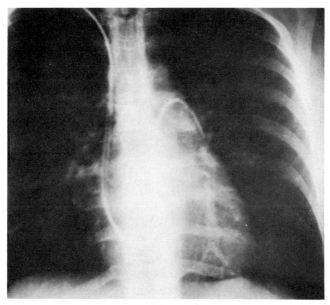

(a)

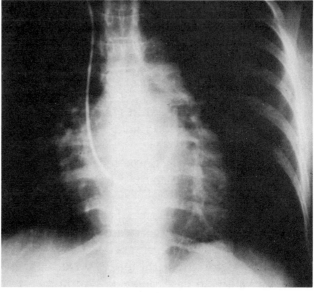

(b)

FIGURE 3.3 *(Continued.)* (c) the Catheter is Now Shown in the Right Lower Lobe Wedge Position; (d) Showing Catheter in the Right Pulmonary Artery. *(Photos Courtesy of Alexander P. Ormond, Jr., Cardiologist.)*

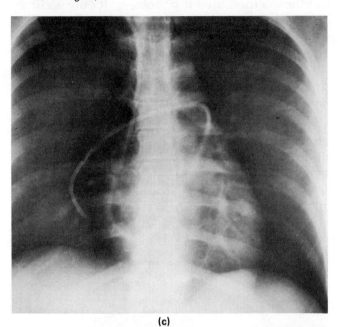

(c)

(d)

ness or nausea, sometimes chilliness and fever. These last only a few hours. After my first catheterization, I was home several hours when I became sick again. A day's rest and the assurances of the doctor ended the problem. It only occurred this one time. My third time went especially well. After the catheterization, I was returned to my room, where I rested for a couple of hours. There were almost no after-symptoms to speak of.

Following the catheterization, the results of the test are analyzed. The findings are explained to you, usually on the next day, along with the doctor's recommendations. For me this was done by Dr. Ormond. He talked to me alone the first time, and then, since my wife was due to visit later in the day, he arranged his schedule to come back and talk to both of us. His report was not unexpected, but it was still a shock; no one is ever really prepared for bad news.

4

THE
BAD
NEWS

Dr. Ormond's findings in both the first catheterization and the third one are quoted below in his own words. His comments help explain what happened after the first operation and why a second operation became necessary. They also explain why it was considered essential to shift the second operation to the Cleveland Clinic Foundation. Furthermore, they add precision and meaning to the history I have been recounting that I, as a layman, am not capable of giving.

Mr. Reinfeld was first seen in February 1975, at which time he had been complaining of pains in the chest which were typical of the pains which occur when the heart does not get enough oxygen. This is called angina pectoris. He would have pressure in the chest with exertion, and it would be relieved by rest. Physical examination at that time was quite unremarkable, but his electrocardiogram and then a stress test were abnormal, which indicated that the heart was not getting enough blood. As a result, it was felt that further testing should be done. This test was to take the form of a heart catheterization to obtain information regarding the degree of blockage in the coronary arteries. Initial catheterization was done in March 1975; this showed complete blockage of the right coronary artery close to where it originated. The distal portion of this vessel was getting some oxygen through a system of collateral vessels. These collaterals form within the body in response to the blockage and provide an auxiliary means of circulation to the area beyond the blockage. The left coronary artery was also blocked, but not completely. At the same time, the main coronary, which divides into two branches, was 50 percent narrowed ahead of the branch. One of the branches appeared to be normal, and the other was 40 to 50 percent blocked.

At this point it appeared that the most viable alternative for the patient was to get more blood to the heart. To do this required a coronary bypass graft. This was done on March 26, 1975, at Akron City Hospital. A bypass graft was constructed to the right coronary artery and also to the anterior descending branch of the left coronary artery. The new blood flow, which can be measured through these bypass grafts, was 40 to 45 cc per minute. This is only moderately good. Postoperatively the patient developed a severe gastric upset due to some medication, but his course was otherwise unremarkable. He was discharged on April 5, 1975, and ordered to take some medicine and gradually to increase his activity.

In August 1975 Mr. Reinfeld began to complain of some pressure in the chest when he would walk and a sensation of filling up inside. While in Amarillo, Texas, in September 1975 he had severe pain and was hospitalized but was told that he did not have any damage to his heart. When I next saw him in 1976 his electrocardiogram was normal, but I felt that he needed further evaluation because of the pains. In March 1976 he returned to my office for an exercise stress test. During the test, he developed pain in the chest, and changes on the electrocardiogram indicated that his heart was not getting enough oxygen. I recommended another catheterization in order to evaluate the status of the bypass grafts and also the status of the native circulation. This was done in August 1976, and at that time it was found that both of the bypass grafts were blocked. This type of blocking occurs in about 10 percent of the cases and probably relates to the low blood flow that occurred through the bypass grafts at the time of the initial operation. However, the native circulation appeared to be unchanged from the year before. At this point new medication was started in an effort to prevent any further pains. He was started on Inderal, which is known to be very effective in preventing angina pectoris. For the next several months Mr. Reinfeld continued to have some pains, but they were rather minimal and did not seem to be increasing in frequency or severity. He would get the pain only if he would overexert himself. I saw him only infrequently during the next several years because he was living in California, but he continued to take the medication faithfully and only rarely required nitroglycerin for his pains. In June 1980 another stress test was done in order to evaluate how he was doing. He achieved a relatively high level of exertion and had some changes in the ECG tracing, but these were not marked and were certainly not worse than the previous tracing.

In May 1981 the pains were thought to have increased a little in severity, but they were not disabling and the medication was continued. There was a pattern of increasing pains until November 1981, when for some reason they stopped completely, for about two weeks. In late November he developed severe chest pain and had to be admitted to the hospital. His electrocardiograms were unchanged, and there was no evidence of new damage to the heart. At this time, because of the increasing pains and this severe episode, I felt that a repeat catheterization was indicated. On December 3, 1981, he underwent his third such procedure. It showed severe blockage in the arteries, much worse than at the time of his catheterization in 1976. The main left coronary was now almost completely blocked, creating a life-threatening situation. As a result, I felt that it was urgent that he undergo a repeat operation, or he would continue to have severe pain and possibly a life-threatening heart attack. I advised that he go to the Cleveland Clinic because of their extensive experience in performing operations on patients who have had previous surgery. The films of the catheterization were sent to Dr. Sheldon at the Cleveland Clinic, and shortly thereafter the patient was admitted for surgery.

These notes from Dr. Ormond are priceless for their simplicity and honesty. But as the victim, I wasn't quite ready for reality, as you will see.

When Dr. Ormond came into my room the day after the catheterization, he seated himself on the edge of the bed. I was sitting in the chair. He discussed what he had found in the tests. He concluded with the statement, "These tests indicate that you need a second operation."

His manner seemed to be brusque and unfeeling, and I resented it. The news was a shock to me, because somehow I was convinced he should have pulled some miracle drug out of his sleeve, like he had been doing over the past five years. Then everything would be normal again. Frankly, I didn't want another operation. I hadn't liked the first one, and I didn't want a second one just like it. I'd had a gallbladder operation fifteen years earlier that hurt much worse, but gallbladders are a dime a dozen compared to hearts.

I began to question his judgment. He said it should be done right away; that I was 95 percent plugged up in the main artery feeding the left side of my heart. Unlike many other parts of the body, if this artery plugged up completely, there would be no other source of supply. I would be dead.

I didn't feel that bad. "Why can't I wait till spring?" I asked, playing for time. Next spring I could stall again, I thought hopefully. But he stood firm, and his voice seemed to me to become angry. I became angry also, perhaps because I felt embarrassed at my own futile tactics. I wanted him to agree with me but also to be honest. I didn't want to die on the basis of my own decision. I wanted him to have that responsibility. But I wanted him to give me a few months to think about it. I just wanted him to back me up and agree with me.

I appreciate now the terribly difficult job doctors have in dealing with critically ill patients. Cardiologists, perhaps more than any other kind of doctor, never meet their patients until they are seriously ill. They seldom grow old together, because so many of their patients are living on borrowed time.

And yet Dr. Ormond was offering me an extension of time that was far safer than I could get by returning home. He was offering me another five or six years, and maybe more, plus improved health, and I resented it. I wanted an easier solution. Instead, he laid it on the line and stubbornly stood his ground. No wonder the doctors who are the most human and compassionate find it hardest to present the facts to their patients. Dr. Ormond and I had, over the space of those short and hurried visits in the past few years, learned to like and respect each other. I was now taking advantage of that personal bond we had built.

When I saw his firmness, I gave in, but I asked once more to at least wait until after Christmas—less than a month away. But again he said it couldn't wait. By now I was really angry and disgusted at his intransigent attitude.

I finally agreed to go ahead without delay. Then he hit me with another setback: He wanted the operation done in Cleveland. He said he had discussed the films with Dr. John Hansel, my previous heart surgeon, and they both felt that this operation required techniques—as you know from Dr. Ormond's notes—not available in Akron.

To me, this was really upsetting. I didn't know anybody at the Cleveland Clinic. I knew the clinic had a good reputation and that patients came to them from all over the world. One of them had been the king of Saudi Arabia. But I had also heard rumors that they used green doctors who operated under the supervision of an expert. The Akron Hospital may have had its faults, but I felt a sense of security there that came from personal contact and prior experience. Besides, I had been happy with Dr. Hansel. I liked his record. I asked Dr. Ormond if he would come up and make hospital calls, and he answered impatiently, "That won't be possible. I have other patients who are very sick and need me." I knew he put in long hours, but I needed a security blanket, even at the expense of his other patients. By now I was almost crying. I didn't even like the idea of my wife having to drive to Cleveland from Akron. The trip took about an hour in good weather, and we were getting into the snowy season. The trip also required driving through the Hough area of Cleveland, where the race riots had occurred fifteen years earlier. The Cleveland Clinic seemed like the worst of all possible choices.

But I agreed, reluctantly, and Dr. Ormond said he would call the clinic and make arrangements to have me admitted.

Next day, I was released to go home on standby until I heard from the clinic.

Dr. Ormond sent the x-ray films and a copy of my file by special courier to Dr. William Sheldon, chairman of the Department of Cardiology at the clinic. After studying the file, the clinic advised that they concurred with Dr. Ormond's analysis and recommendations. While I was waiting to hear from the clinic, Dr. Ormond called me several evenings to see how things were going. A week after leaving City Hospital, I checked into the clinic. This week of waiting was an important one for me, as it was also for others with similar problems.

One of the patients I met at the clinic, while I was recovering from the operation, had had his most harrowing experience during this period. This man had a bad heart valve. Even during the most sedentary activity, such as watching TV at home, without notice his lungs would begin to fill with fluid and he'd start choking for breath. As a consequence, on the day before he was to be admitted to the clinic, he developed pneumonia, and the operation had to be postponed until he recovered.

In my own case, that week was a period to adjust my thinking and to become resigned to my fate. It was also a chance for my daughter Carol to practice the nursing profession at home. I had her remove the stitches from my arm and saved a trip to the doctor's office. I was still mad at Dr. Ormond. I don't know what he had done wrong, but I was still angry enough that I was seriously thinking of switching doctors after my operation.

I don't know how many other patients get mad at their doctors for telling the truth, but I suspect that it happens often. Steve McQueen, the actor, comes to mind, with his sad but fruitless search for a miracle cure for cancer. Other accounts I have read tell of people who have searched the world over for an escape from reality, but in the long run there is no escape. Unfortunately, both the patient and the doctor pay a price. It's not fair to the doctor, and if the patient runs until he finds a doctor who tells him what he wants to hear, it's the patient who ultimately pays for his folly.

During this period, I kept all my bills paid up to the day, so that my wife wouldn't have to worry about missing a payment. I went over them with her and listed on a sheet of paper all the payments and due dates she should be aware of for such things as our home and insurances and other long-term commitments. I also made up a list of instructions on where to find records. We discussed moving to an apartment with less responsibility and fewer expenses if something happened to me. We discussed my son Nick's going to college. We tried to cover everything, so that my wife would have a grasp of the business and our financial operations if tragedy struck. This was one of the advantages of the warning we got that many others do not get. When death strikes suddenly, there is no planning together, no period of preparation. As it happened, we didn't need it, but blessings resulted from it all nevertheless.

I'm reminded here of the title of this chapter, "The Bad News." When I showed the outline of this book to Mrs. Danni Nadler, R.N., cardiovascular counselor at the clinic, the first remark she made was with regard to the name of the chapter: "Bad news?" she said. "I would think it was good news." She was right, of course. I hadn't been threatened. I'd been given a reprieve. I know that now, but I didn't feel that way at the time.

When I went to the clinic, I wasn't very certain I was going to survive. I had gone through this once. My condition was more serious than before. The operation also was more of a threat, and I was six years older. The chance of failure was greater. Those were the indisputable facts, and apparently it was all Dr. Ormond's fault. No wonder I was mad at him.

5

THOUGHTS
WHILE AWAITING
THE OPERATION

Hospitals,
Government,
and Bureaucracy

During that long week or so that I was waiting to hear from the clinic, my mind traveled over a lot of problems—as the mind does when the body is physically inactive and the future is foreshortened. There was a big void of uncertainty ahead. The operation offered no guarantees, only probabilities: Beyond lay death, or perhaps disablement; or, if the gods smiled upon me once more, a new lease on life. President Carter may have been born again; a cat may have nine lives; but for me, I was about to try for my third. This in itself is a unique phenomenon that few have experienced so clearly as I: For me, the date of rebirth and revitalization can be fixed accurately.

For the born-again Christian there is an oozing in of the spirit, an osmotic flow in which the individual gradually becomes aware of the change. He is born again by a transition in his life, even though he becomes aware of the presence of God and Christ suddenly. It is this moment of awareness for which he declares himself reborn. But the cat never heard of the legend, and there is no formal renewal of life. For the heart patient, however, the operation is the ultimate reality. There is a precise sense of finality. It is both exciting and fearful to contemplate. Like the battlefield, it is man's greatest arena, and his greatest threat. If he survives, his outlook on life has changed. He is more human. More tolerant. More concerned with people. If he dies, of course, it's over. But it's over neatly. There is no long dragged-out pain and suffering. To die while under the anesthesia has its compensations, which are not entirely undesirable or disturbing. There is no pain, once you're out, which is far better than you have facing you if you survive. That is why, in the first sentence of chapter 2, I said I didn't know whether to be "frightened or relieved."

Heart patients are probably luckier than most, because death is seldom postponed. It seldom offers you long periods of agony and suffering, as happens with so many other diseases. Some diseases terrify me much more. There's a certain

51

comfort in knowing you will probably "pop" out of this world suddenly some day. (I hope they don't beat on my chest like they do on TV!) In the meantime, you can live a somewhat normal life, thanks to modern medicine. When you're ready for the bed, you're also ready for the grave. Thank heaven. To me this is important. It is also important to others, as I have learned from close friends. One friend of over twenty-five years asked me to promise not to let him suffer with a terminal illness but to put him out of his misery if he cannot lift his own hand. What could I answer? He promised me the same consideration. He has made the request several times. I hope, and expect, I will never need it. Hence, there is some comfort, as well as deep concern, with the heart problem. As I say, we may be the lucky ones.

There is another concern with the heart operation. The patient can have a stroke during the operation, so it is possible to suffer debilitation of a permanent nature. Such occurrences are rare, but they are a threat that must be acknowledged.

A week of lying around with a crisis-stimulated mind opens up all sorts of avenues for thought. TV doesn't enchant me, and radio only captures the aural part of the mind. In some respects, music stimulates the mind, so that it can have both pleasures at once, each sense idling in unison.

My mind returned to that room at the hospital. I know that to some extent my reaction had been brought on by my state of mind, my dejection. But I had noticed other things. In previous trips to the hospital there was always a certain sense of guilt or shame, like I had let my family down or failed them.

Attending this was an added sense of being stripped of my dignity. In the hospital you wear gowns and are reduced to the status of a number. A friend, Vernon Oldham, who is a patent attorney, made almost this identical remark to me over lunch one day. So much emphasis is placed on physical recovery that the human element is allowed to suffer. The physical condition of the room is symptomatic of the total psychological problem facing the patient.

And yet, isn't the inner man also in need of food and nourishment? Isn't the spiritual and artistic man important in the curing process, so that the one cannot proceed without the other? Haven't these hospitals heard the old proverb "A merry heart doeth good like a medicine"?

Set aside for the moment the spiritual needs of the patient as expressed in his relationship to God. There is also an inner need for assurance that comes from his senses and surroundings—aesthetic qualities, perhaps. Both of these areas are of vital interest not only to the patient but to the hospital as well, because they affect the attitude and confidence of the patient. They influence his chances and rate of recovery. If 90 percent of all illness is psychosomatic, as some claim, then for some patients this may be the most important ingredient in the cure.

We all develop a normal level of expectancy that we strive for in our home. Do we not have a right to find this or better in our new home as well? The transfer from home to hospital should be an uplifting experience in every way possible, to offset the shock and dismay that attend the circumstances. A hospital visit is not a vacation junket, but it need not ignore the possibilities.

When I travel and stay in a hotel, I pick places that are above or equal to my status in life. I like hotels that feature exterior landscaping and decorator-designed interiors— places that are exciting and are available to me only for a moment. I like to feel that this is one of the benefits of travel. It is one of the "perks" of business that makes an otherwise dismal experience worthwhile and endurable. In like manner, when I vacation, like most people, I seek to recreate, to surround myself with the pleasures of nature and the gifts of man, even if only for a fleeting period of time.

In this respect I think we do more for the dead than the living. We would never, for instance, haul our dead to the grave in a pine box in the back of an old pickup truck. It might be cheaper, but we cannot bring ourselves to it. Instead, we honor the dead with chauffeur-driven Cadillacs and satin-lined coffins. No bulldozer is used to cover a gunny-sacked body thrown in a trench. Instead, we put a suit on the corpse —perhaps the only one he ever wore—and bury it with its rings and gold inlays, items he might need in heaven, I presume. We raise the dead to a status higher than he ever had in life. This is the moment when we are most vulnerable to predatory funeral practices, because we want the best for those about whom we cared the very most.

If these costly manifestations are so important to the dead, are they less important to the living? Can't our sick and dying be treated as well? Not everyone is so sick that one cannot appreciate one's surroundings; and even when one is very sick, there may be moments, even if unspoken or unconsciously observed, when one smiles inwardly.

As I reflect on what I have just written, it becomes obvious that I was not just upset by the physical surroundings at the hospital but that something else was ticking away in my brain. The mental conditions of humanity and the *merry hearts* of the patients are obviously important, but these I can leave to the professionals who get their chance at us later. The truth is, now that it's out on the table, it's the bill that was bothering me—the costs I was going to have to pay for all this care I was about to receive. Like eating in a plush restaurant on my own expenses, I didn't know whether to enjoy myself or not, whether I should appreciate the attention or resent it.

Frankly, hospital bills always seem too high, when I get them, and if they had to be paid in advance, I might be tempted to pass the opportunity along to a later date.

How these bills are arrived at has always been a mystery to me that defieth understanding. They seem to make no sense at all. All I know is that they increase in geometrical proportion with time, for no apparent reason. Therefore, being of sound mind and of questionable body, I resolved to get to the bottom of this mystery. This meant doing some sleuthing on my own, which I couldn't do yet because, as you'll remember, I was sick. So I decided to check it out later, after I had recovered. I tucked the questions away in my bosom and promised myself to get the facts as soon as I could think straight. Since there's some question as to whether that would ever happen, I waited only until the bills came rolling in and then decided to seek my revenge, to strike back and land a blow for the little man—all of us helpless victims of society and social cancer.

There can be no secret to the fact that hospital and medical costs are rising rapidly. These conclusions are supported by well-established statistics published directly by the Department of Health and Human Services (formerly the Department of Health, Education, and Welfare). For example, in 1940 the total per-capita expenditure for health in the U.S. was $29.62 per year. In 1965 it was $210.89. By 1970 this figure had risen to $357.90. In 1975 it was $603.57, in 1979 it was $936.92, and in 1980 it was $1067.06. (These figures are projected by the department to exceed $3000 by 1990!)

From 1930 until 1970, medical costs were doubling almost every ten years. Then, from 1970 on, health care expenditures took an upswing, tripling in less than nine years. National health expenditures grew at a compound rate of 13 percent between 1973 and 1979. When these figures are adjusted for inflation, however, the rate of increase in constant (noninflated) dollars averaged 4.4 percent during these years.

Physician's charges increased at a slightly lower rate than that of hospitals and drugs. In 1965, for example, they amounted to $43 per person, and in 1979 they averaged $180 per person—a growth of 420 percent. This compares with a growth of 445 percent for all costs, including hospitals and drugs.

It is hard to begrudge these people, who have given one third of their productive lives to study and research, anything they can reasonably earn. The doctors I know—perhaps I've been fortunate—are dedicated men and women. I may wince at times when I get their bills, but when I consider their incomes in the light of the earnings of other professional groups—who have neither the responsibilities nor the pressures, around the clock—I do not envy them. I would not trade them place for place nor dollar for dollar.

In 1981, for example, the top twenty-one executives in the greater Akron metropolitan area earned salaries and bonuses ranging from $120,086 to $835,969. These men were presidents or chairmen of manufacturing firms, banks, drug firms, utilities, and trucking companies. Their responsibilities and commitments were great. But none of them was responsible for actual life and death. For a doctor, these are decisions that must be made daily.

The average gross income for a physician in 1978 was $111,900.[1] Net income from the medical practice, after office expenses and help, was $65,500. When these figures are adjusted for inflation over the preceding ten years, however, the physician actually earned $33,487 *before taxes* in 1968 dollars. These figures compare to a net income in 1968 of $35,866, so that your doctor's income has actually been declining at the rate of 1 percent per year since 1968! Making matters even worse, every doctor has been in the same boat as the rest of us who pay taxes. Physicians' taxes have arched higher because of inflation, so that their "take-home pay" has declined even more.

The amount that inflation has added to the cost of medical care is shown in Fig. 5.1. The term *changes in intensity* refers to the increase in the number of benefits provided by current medical care facilities and physicians. Population growth is included because the expenditure figures given at the right of the graph are total national expenditures rather than the amount spent on a per-capita basis. The most important point is that inflation represents almost three fourths of the increase in health care costs.

Unfortunately, the problem of medical costs does not end with inflation. As with any type of industry, total medical care costs should decline with time. Operations that took two hours should take one hour with practice, new skills, and new equipment. Hence, costs should decline, but they don't. Instead they have been increasing.

There are several factors that can be blamed for this, the least of which are greed and lack of compassion. The most common of these factors are those that involve "administrative and bureaucratic" costs, as we shall see.

Unfortunately, the problem with hospital costs is that many of them are influenced by outside sources. It is hard to appreciate how much the social changes of the past forty years have influenced these costs. We sometimes do not realize, for example, that we have a government that both giveth and

[1] See American Medical Association, *Profile of Medical Practice* (AMA Center for Health Services Research and Development, 1980), and U.S. Department of Human Services, *Health Care Financing Review,* Winter 1981 (Washington, D.C.: U.S. Government Printing Office).

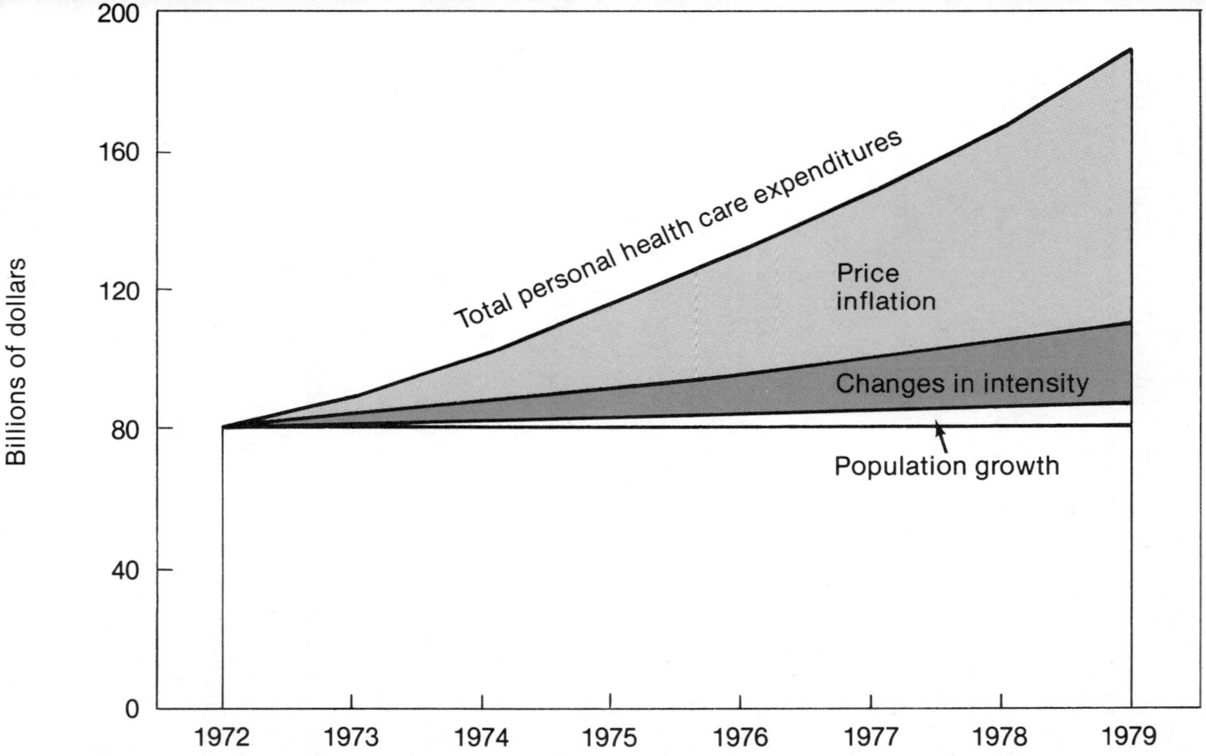

FIGURE 5.1 Sources of Growth in Personal Health Care Expenditures, 1972–1979. (*Robert M. Gibson, "National Health Expenditures, 1979,"* Health Care Financing Review, *Summer 1980.*)

taketh away. Like so many charities, the administrative costs of government have become so great that the part that it giveth is exceeded greatly by the part that it taketh.

Because I am closer to the situation in industry than in the non-profit arena I will demonstrate this with an illustration taken there first, but the point being made will be clear enough.

In the state of Ohio, the sales tax on all manufactured products sold to the public is 5 percent of total sales. On products such as autos the resale price is also taxed. Furthermore, retail stores usually mark up goods 100 percent, so that the Ohio sales tax based on the manufacturer's price averages close to 10 percent on all manufactured goods! These figures do not include corporate or personal income taxes or fees that the state also gets. Now, corporate profits in a typical year in the United States, for the past decade, have averaged about 5 percent on sales, according to government figures. Since these are after-tax figures, the federal government has already taken a share roughly equal to this amount, plus taxes on the people who work at the plants, and also taxes on any profits remitted to the stockholders. In all, the various governments get almost five times as much as the man who risks his money to run the plant. The government gets its share at no risk and no investment.

But this is not where the problem begins. The problem springs from the number of reports and records that are required. Because the government cannot trust the taxpayers, it builds up large bureaucracies to audit and see that the rules and regulations are enforced. Industry in turn finds that it needs a similar force to defend itself and provide the information sought by the bureaucracy. The result is a form of decay that breeds upon itself.

Perhaps the first to sense this type of encroachment were the Romans, 1700 years ago.

Roughly four decades before Constantine became the first Christian emperor, Lactantius tells us that the number of those on the state payroll (and dole) was larger than the number of taxpayers. He was probably exaggerating because he was a Christian and the emperor was not. But we have his word for it. In more modern times, we have volumes of figures

THOUGHTS WHILE AWAITING THE OPERATION

to show what happens to a country, and our conclusions need not be left to impressions.

One of the first formal studies of the growth of bureaucracy was that of C. Northcote Parkinson. Parkinson stated the growth he observed as a form of natural law which now bears his name. He observed that work simply expands to fill the time available. Thus, long before the Falkland Islands became a battleground in 1982, he had discovered that the "magnificent Navy on land" of the British was much more in evidence than that which put out to sea. The sea navy, with which Britain had ruled the waves, was in eclipse. From 1914 to 1928, for example, it had declined one third in seamen and two thirds in ships (from 146,000 officers and men in 1914 to 100,000 in 1928). The land navy, made up of admiralty officials, on the other hand, was in robust health, having increased 78 percent. Since single examples do not stand very well alone, he gave us another, this time from the records of the colonial office. It seems that from 1935 to 1954, during which the British territories were in steady decline, the number of administrative officials increased almost fivefold.

Parkinson did not study our own country, fortunately, sparing us the embarrassment, but the situation is quite similar. Our Navy of 1982 had 464 ships in commission and 4867 captains. During World War II, the Navy had 5718 ships and 3876 captains.

These types of problems seem to happen to everybody. For example, in our rubber plants in Akron, workers work six hours and get paid for eight. The Los Angeles *Herald Examiner* made a study of refuse collectors in 1978 that showed that the average driver and loader worked only five hours out of eight. Furthermore, when the workload increased, as it did in summer, instead of working a full schedule, the new demands were met by hiring seventy more crews, who were kept in reserve to meet these needs.

In Ohio, the population has not varied since 1970, but state employment has increased 32 percent. The city of Akron, on the other hand, since 1940 has actually lost 20 percent of its population. Where once stood a single administrative building in 1940, there now stands double the office space, a five-story federal building and a state building have been added, and plans are afoot, as I write this, for a fifteen-story state office tower.

Just the week I penned these notes, I stopped in at the auto license bureau to transfer a title. In a room with close to fifty desks, less than half were attended at any one time. Where were the other people? In the twenty minutes or so that I was there, some came and went, but at no time were more than half working at once.

This bureaucratic growth extends far wider than only those areas affected by the tax auditing. It includes, in fact, all those activities in which the government shows an interest, in which it seeks information or exerts influence. Senator John Glenn called government paperwork "the biggest hidden tax in America." He said that in 1979 businesses filed 305 million forms and *answered 7.3 billion questions,* at an estimated cost of $103 billion. Naturally, the government is interested in protecting its interests, and to do this it must set up rules and standards.

The government's interest and influence, therefore, in an area or sector of society are directly proportionate to the amount of funds that flow between it and the sector involved.

Local and state governments have always played some role in regional hospital activities—establishing minimum standards and acceptable operating rules, for example—but these roles have been limited and distant. But within our lifetime, since World War II, the federal government has become actively engaged in health care and funding, with the result that there has been a large increase in regulations and reporting.

In 1950 federal health expenditures were $1.6 billion and state and local expenditures were $1.8 billion. In other words, they were roughly the same. This relative balance remained until 1965. Thereafter, the federal government's share increased rapidly, so that by 1970 the federal share was $17.7 billion and state and local was $10.1 billion. Both had increased rapidly, under federal stimulation and prodding, but the federal share was almost double that of state and local share. By 1980 the federal government, through its Medicare and Medicaid plans, was pumping $71 billion into the medical system, and the state-local share was $33 billion. Together these funds represented almost 40 percent of our national health bill.

The purpose and compassion represented by these government efforts are commendable and beyond question. But the results have been far less satisfactory than the casual observer would expect as seen under the microscope of cold statistics. (As we already know, the government does not "give" without imposing a heavy burden upon the receiver.)

The unusual result of the government's increased intervention into the medical field was to pump up the cost.

Here again, the government itself is our best source of information.

Health Care Financing Review for September 1981 pointed out, for example, that "the most notable aspect of health care spending in 1980 was its accelerated growth. The 15.2 percent increase in overall health expenditures is the highest in the last 15 years. . . . This increase occurred at a time when the overall economy grew by 8.8 percent. Thus, the share of the GNP (Gross National Product) occupied by health care spending spurted from 8.9 percent in 1979 to 9.4 percent in 1980."[2]

Prior to this, the spring 1980 issue of the same periodical warned that "research has shown that even with an increase in Federal program fees, the Medicare and Medicaid recipients may not have greater access to care. Hadley and Lea (1978) and Paringer (1979) report that raising Medicare and Medicaid fees might exert inflationary pressures on private levels, leaving the relative positions of the fees in the private and public sectors the same as before the increase."[3]

This article points out that special tax concessions have led to inefficient administration of some insurance plans, compared to plans that receive no tax advantages. The authors' own studies show that nonprofit insurance plans such as Blue Cross and Blue Shield, with tax advantages over private for-profit plans, did *"not reduce* premium levels but

[2] Robert M. Gibson and Daniel R. Waldo, "National Health Expenditures, 1980," *Health Care Financing Review,* September 1981, p. 3.

[3] Nancy Greenspan and Ronald J. Vogel, "Taxation and Its Effect upon Public and Private Health Insurance and Medical Demand," *Health Care Financing Review,* Spring 1980, p. 39.

instead lent to higher fees and excess administrative costs." As the government has increased its efforts to help the public, the benefits have been wiped out by the increased paperwork burden.

The authors conclude by saying that the inefficiencies created by the tax subsidies for the buyers and sellers of health insurance provide evidence "that the present tax structure of the private health industry contributes to the rising costs in the medical care sector."[4]

Hence, direct aid in terms of Medicare and Medicaid and indirect aid in terms of tax subsidies have both combined to exert upward pressures on prices that have tended to nullify the benefits they were intended to provide.

An indirect factor that has also contributed to the steady increase in medical costs has been the courts.

Through its policies of liberal interpretations of personal liabilities, the courts of the United States have made our country the most litigious society since the Periclean days of Athens. The United States has nearly 600,000 registered lawyers, of whom 30,000 make their home in Washington, D.C.; the whole country of Japan supports only 12,000 lawyers.

Because the courts cannot accurately distinguish between unscrupulous, opportunistic claims and justifiable damages, the number of malpractice suits in the United States has increased dramatically in this decade, creating substantial costs for the profession (and therefore the patient). It is no surprise, therefore, to find that the most rapidly increasing category of costs in the medical field is for malpractice insurance. During the nine-year period, from 1970 to 1978, the costs of malpractice insurance increased at an annual rate of 39 percent. In other words, these costs, which are borne by the hospital and the physician out of necessity, were almost doubling every year and a half. In fact, in 1975 they doubled in a single year. Naturally, these costs are passed on to the patient. At the present time, the current rate that the profession is paying for this type of insurance adds almost 4 percent to the total medical bill. I estimate that my own share of this cost alone was almost $1000! In other words, my open heart opera-

---

[4] Ibid., p. 43.

tion, which cost about $25,000 from inception of the second illness until the six week checkup after surgery included almost $1000 to cover the insurance premium needed to protect the medical profession should I sue later and win a court settlement.

These claims for damages are not limited to the medical profession but are widespread throughout our society. In the farm implement business, for example, product liability insurance premiums often exceed the total profits of the manufacturer. Twenty-five years ago, this type of coverage was rare and inexpensive. Today, these forms of insurance are often required by law, under the umbrella of consumer protection.

If these examples were taken at random, it might be argued that they are not representative of the true situation. But such is not the case. The next fastest growing area of cost in hospitals is for employee benefits, another area heavily influenced by government intervention. At 19 percent per year, these costs, adjusted for inflation, are growing at a rate more than double that of other medical costs.

Payroll expenses and employee benefits represent almost 60 percent of the costs in a hospital.

The number of employees in an activity, as we have seen, is a function of the true work that has to be done, plus the administrative work that is required to meet the special demands of society. The efficiency of a hospital is impaired when its staff is not being utilized to perform the tasks for which it is trained—when the doctors and nurses are diverted from the medical profession into the role of administrators and processors of records. My daughter Carol, who is a registered nurse at one of the largest hospitals in northern Ohio, reports that much of her time is lost this way. She estimates that even as a beginning nurse she spent 30 percent of her time at reports and desk work and that her supervisor spent 100 percent of her time away from actual nursing duties.

The extent to which this trend—this curse of Parkinson—has permeated the industry was pointed up by a report of the American Hospital Association in 1978. In 1960, for example, total hospital employment numbered 114 persons per 100 patients. Seventeen years later, the figure had nearly tripled: It now took 301 persons on the payroll to service 100 patients. Furthermore, these changes do not necessarily imply an improvement in service. As a rule, if the growth of staff follows the pattern of industry, the general effect is to stifle efficiency. There has, in fact, been an actual decline in the utilization of hospital beds during this same period.

Unfortunately, as we have seen in the studies on insurance programs, inefficiencies of administration are more apt to be exacerbated in a charitable institution than in one committed to making a profit.

This does not mean that profit-making corporations have achieved a miraculous cure that the others have missed. Quite the contrary; profit-making corporations are as plagued by the problems of administrative creep as anyone, but they have had more success in containing it, thanks almost entirely to the pressures of the profit motive. In this respect a major incentive to improve is forced upon them with each recession, and cutbacks in office personnel are necessary to survive. The heavy reductions in white-collar workers made by the auto industry in the early eighties finds no parallel in not-for-profit organizations.

Utilities and insurance programs proceed without interruption, through good times and bad, as do most government programs.

The result is that hospitals and charitable organizations tend to accept administrative inefficiencies as part of the price of providing service.

What efforts are made at cost controls are often more visible than actual, and sometimes they show up in unusual ways.

The drabness of the room I mentioned is an example. This is a condition almost indigenous to public facilities in which an outward appearance of frugality seems to be obligatory. Examples are widespread and include employment offices, welfare rooms, state buildings, prisons, classrooms, dorms, and license bureaus.

The great marble domed buildings of the past, built when the country had less money but greater aesthetic appreciation, are no longer an expression of the youthfulness of America. Everything seems old and in need of paint. It is almost as if we no longer care for the spirit but only for the function.

In expressing an appreciation for the aesthetic qualities of man, profit-making organizations have been more effective than their counterparts in the nonprofit sector. Commercial buildings, like hotels and restaurants, for example, depend heavily upon decor for their survival. These include many fast-food chains such as Denny's and Red Lobster, just to name two at random, that are a delight to visit. The surroundings are as attractive as the menus.

We must not be misled into thinking that drabness is synonymous with efficiency. As a rule, most successful firms take great pride in their offices and facilities, using architects and landscapers to achieve an aura of success. As a result, the buildings are interesting and the office decor inspires confidence and an air of accomplishment.

The exceptions usually correlate with the firms that are having problems. My own experiences along these lines may be of interest.

I took over as president of a company a few years ago, and my office was in worse shape than the restrooms. The shades were of the old, pull-down type. They were yellowed with age and tattered at the edges. Papers were loosely stacked in piles on tables and chairs. Beyond meeting the people, my first act as president was to replace the shades with drapes, clean up the papers, and completely redecorate the office. We didn't have a penny to spare, as you know if you read my book *Survival Management,* and we certainly needed money to spend elsewhere more than in the office, but my feelings were that it was not enough to tell people there had been a change in management. It must be visible as well, both to the people on the floor and to our customers and suppliers. Morale and attitude are important factors to success. Our company became profitable in six months.

The point is that morale, attitude, and efficiency must permeate the building, from the top to the bottom. Every employee must sense the purpose and scope of his place in the organization.

To some extent, these demands may seem unfair. I may

be asking too much. But on the other hand, is it really unfair to demand from the medical profession what so many professional administrators have failed to accomplish?

Even the highest-caliber business colleges, which should be more capable than a hospital, for example, do not always operate efficiently. There is an embarrassment of riches, of intelligence and learning, with a dearth of administrative capability. The professional, whether a teacher or a physician, concentrates on his or her craft rather than administration. And this is as we would want it, surely, for any hospital where we'd go. As a result, in recent years, there has been a trend toward professional management in the nonprofit sector of our society—a form of dichotomy between the doer and the administrator. A number of hospitals and colleges that have struggled to provide low-cost benefits to the public have improved their costs and economics through increased use of professional managers. Such moves benefit the medical staffs, the hospitals, and the public, provided there is no decline in quality of service. Quite unexpectedly, service frequently improves when efficient administration spreads over into all areas, freeing doctors and other medical specialists to do the job they are best suited for.

The hospital in Wellington is an example of this developing trend. The Wellington Hospital was run by a retired industrial executive who had moved to a farm in Wellington from Cleveland, where he had chosen to spend the final years of his life. As for all good men who retire, there is no real retirement. Good talent is always in demand. At first he agreed only to help out. But he did such an excellent job that they wouldn't let him quit.

Professional management means introducing sound and effective cost controls, administered by a trained team of managers. It means setting up standards of performance and time standards for completing certain functions.

In searching through the data for this chapter, I was surprised to find that there are published figures showing estimated times for completing various types of operations. These figures are useful guidelines in scheduling facilities and patient flow. If the idea seems unnecessarily risky, keep in mind the fact that there is a very close correlation between skill and output. Life on the operating table itself can very well depend upon the skill and the speed with which the operation is completed.

Major savings are to be had, especially, in those sectors of the hospital where the function is not critical but where inefficient effort can result in delays and dangerous errors, where large numbers of people are engaged in multifarious tasks in support of the main objective.

CONCLUSIONS

In the midst of my studies, I came upon a rather startling disclosure regarding my own experiences. If we take the cost of my first operation and compare it to the cost of my second, in which all conditions were essentially identical, the second operation, after adjusting for inflation, was considerably cheaper!

This is as it should be, of course, if anything has been learned over the past six years. Equipment is better. Techniques are better. Even the process has evolved and improved. Hence, the medical profession does follow the same type of cost curve commonly found in industry when introducing a new product.

It seems, therefore, safe to say that hospitals and the medical profession are passing along the benefits of their learning to the public whenever possible. They are reacting in a competitive way to the natural market forces.

6

ENTERING
THE
CLINIC

It's obvious that many of the thoughts in chapter 5 never even entered my head while I was lying around at home. At best only the seeds were planted there.

Most of my time was spent listening to classical music on the radio or feeling sorry for myself. I rather enjoyed the latter, and by the time the call came from the clinic I was bored enough to look forward to a change. They told me I was to report that next afternoon.

After all the waiting, it was time at last to be doing something.

As I say, my gloom was pretty well dispersed by now, and my mind adjusted to my fate. I was almost eager to go.

My wife Ginny and I left home in late morning the next day. My son was in school and my daughters were involved in their own activities.

My wife, faithfully serving as chauffeur, trundled me through falling snow and blustering wind on the road from Bath to Cleveland. For people who live in big cities, it would have been a normal hour's drive. To me the forty-five miles seemed like a very long trip, isolating me from friends and family.

When we arrived at the clinic, I was pleasantly surprised to find that all my musings about the neglected inner man were only partially correct. Here was an exception.

The clinic had many of the characteristics of a campus, and indeed it was so called by its own people. The "campus" was located on some fifty acres in a heavily urbanized section on the east side of Cleveland. It had originally been founded by a group of four physicians in 1921 and had since grown to become a national health resource, treating patients from throughout the world. The Cleveland Clinic Foundation consists of a clinic, a research division, an education division and a hospital. The clinic handles more than 380,000 patient visits each year, and the hospital provides care for some 32,000

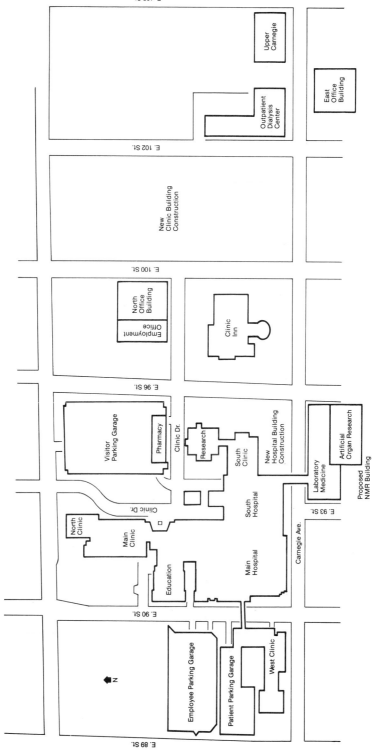

FIGURE 6.1 The Cleveland Clinic Foundation, 9500 Euclid Avenue, Cleveland, Ohio 44106. *(Courtesy of Cleveland Clinic Foundation.)*

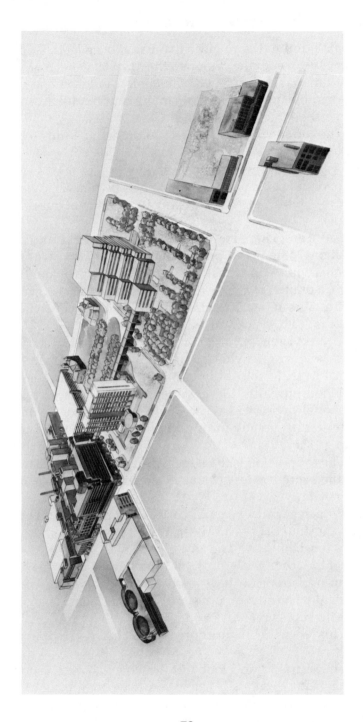

FIGURE 6.1 *(Continued.)*

patients admitted annually. It contains over 1000 beds. Enlargements of both the clinic and the hospital were in progress at the time. When finished, the clinic would be one of the largest ambulatory care centers in the country. It had already become the largest employer in Cleveland.

The foundation treats more children and adults for cancer than any other facility in Ohio.

A layout of the campus is shown in Fig. 6.1. A unique feature of the clinic is that it contains its own hotel, called the Clinic Inn, which provides lodging for families of out-of-town patients.

Services include interpreters (Arabic, French, and Spanish, among others); an ombudsman, to help you with your problems while you are at the clinic; counseling for family and patient; a branch of a major bank; a barber; a travel office; and three restaurants—a cafeteria in the hospital, a coffee house, and a first-rate restaurant in the Inn.

The division of research investigates the mysteries of medical science. Activities range from the development of an artificial heart to the study of hardening of the arteries and high blood pressure. Closely integrated with research is the educational division, which provides continuing education for physicians already in private practice, plus students and others.

The foundation is the largest postgraduate medical facility in the United States not connected with a medical school or university.

With regard to heart disease, the nation's number one killer, the foundation has been the site of pioneering techniques for diagnosing and treating the disease. The development of the coronary bypass, the arteriogram, and new drugs to treat hypertension have probably saved millions of lives worldwide. Foundation physicians and surgeons have one of the best success records in the world.

This was the institution to which I had committed myself.

The entrance and lobby to the hospital were tastefully and colorfully decorated. The furniture was of the quality of a Hilton or Hyatt hotel. Because we arrived at noon, we tried the cafeteria and found it bright and cheerful. It could compete in decor with the best of the quick-food restaurants. The food, unfortunately, was mediocre, but it was edible if you chose your portions carefully. (We did not try the other restaurants, even later.)

Nor was the theme abandoned at the elevator door. Upstairs, the hallways, corridors, and wards were crisp and neat. The signs of decay, of which I had spoken earlier, were not apparent here. For me, at least, there was a sense of efficiency and quality that gave me encouragement and assurance. You must remember that as of this moment, I had not yet met any of the doctors in whose hands I would be placing my life; the impression I received on entering the clinic played a vital role in my attitude toward and acceptance of the events of the next ten days. I am a snob at heart, as you have noticed, probably unkindly, and I feel closer to God in a beautiful cathedral than in a simple abode. The preacher may be quite mediocre, but he has a tremendous head start with me when he expounds his preachings surrounded by awesome beauty.

Such are the attitudes of the mind, which no doubt make no sense in heaven. I will probably be called upon to justify this narrow-mindedness when I eventually get there, if ever. These continual postponements, which keep delaying my arrival, however, lead me to suspect that it will be some time off. (There may come a time when I will, in fact, resent these miraculous postponements and will say "No more!"; for now, I'm happy with each extension.)

When I walked up to the admitting desk, I had expected to go straight to my room. Instead there were the usual delays on checking in, and I became impatient. Perhaps it was the reality of the situation that overwhelmed me and made me fret. More likely, I was disturbed by the idea of waiting, much as people fret at a slow-moving car blocking their way, even when they know that to hurry only means more waiting later. I have always had trouble fitting myself into other people's shoes. Somehow it seemed to me that they ought to move faster or get out of the way. Delays always upset me and make me irritable. I'm the perfect Type A personality, the classic textbook example of a person who develops heart problems. This interminable waiting wasn't helping a bit.

When I reached the desk, the receptionist took my name

and told me to have a seat in the waiting area and that she would call me. My wife and I chose a comfortable spot on a couch and began looking for reading matter. From years of training we had come to expect old issues of weekly news magazines, such as *Time* and *U.S. News.* These are standard fare at doctor's and dentist's offices, as you know. Either current issues get stolen, or the good issues, like *Playboy,* circulate among the licentious staff members before they reach the waiting room. By the time the patient gets them they are like yesterday's newspapers. The good pictures are removed. Occasionally I have sat in waiting rooms with *National Geographic* or other equally timeless material.

When we sat down, we were surprised to find that there were no magazines at all. Someone must have stolen them I thought. I looked around for the thief, figuring he would have a stack of magazines stuffed under his arm, no doubt stashed in a corner, hiding them, greedily reading in privacy. But there was no one in sight to fit the description. In fact, there were no magazines at all. There weren't even any three months later when I returned to the scene of the crime to gather information for these notes. Either the thief had returned once more, just ahead of me, or the clinic couldn't afford magazines. The only things available were newspapers from a coin dispenser. Well, that was better than old magazines anyway, I thought, so I bought a paper and read it. I could have read half a dozen before they called me.

When they did, I was directed to the credit department. Here, anticipating my thoughts, the credit manager, a very stern and suspicious woman, reviewed my insurance policy and asked me if I had the money to pay my bill. She couldn't have read my notes because I hadn't written them yet. It must have been something about my manner. Then she called the insurance company, to see if they were solvent or still existed.

Finally, when she was satisfied that I wasn't there under false pretenses, trying to get a free operation, she directed me to the second floor so I could meet my doctor.

The second floor was like the waiting room to a typical doctor's office. In fact, it was the lobby for a number of doctors. It was here that I discovered that all doctor's offices are the same everywhere in the world. It was here that all those missing magazines were! I have rechecked my facts by returning here, several times since, and I can state in all honesty that not one magazine was less than four months old! As it turns out, this is almost exactly the time lag that your insurance company is going to take to part with its check to pay the clinic. At least mine took this long, or longer, and this may explain the suspicious credit manager. Is it possible for there to be a correlation between the age of the magazines in the waiting room and the age of the bill?

Up on the second floor, for the first time, I met Dr. Leonard Golding, the surgeon who was going to perform the operation. Dr. Golding outlined the basic plan to both my wife and me and mentioned that three to four bypasses would be made, depending on what turned up after they looked inside. The operation was scheduled for 7 A.M. on the morning of December 18. This gave me two days to relax and adapt to the hospital. Dr. Golding was a pleasant fellow and answered our questions patiently. Like Dr. Hansel, he had the long slim fingers expected of a surgeon, and then to top it off, after we left his office, my wife remarked how handsome he was!

With these two recommendations going for him, I knew I had another winner in Dr. Golding. It certainly made the rest of my day. Rest assured that if I ever go through this again, I will be most leary of any surgeon who has either short, fat fingers or about whom my wife should remark, "My, wasn't he homely?"

As it was, I was so delighted with my good fortune in being assigned to Dr. Golding that I completely forgot to check out his batting average. It may not have been as meaningful in my case as it was the first time. Second-timers, who have been through the operation before, don't always do as well as those on their first trip. They have more complications and special problems. It may have been just as well that I didn't ask. As I found out later, in talking to others at the hospital, Dr. Golding was one of the best on the staff.

Remember this, then, in choosing your own surgeon: He must have long slim fingers and my wife must think he's good looking. If he doesn't meet these two scientific criteria, especially the latter, you are on your own. You will probably do just as well as I have done—I sincerely expect so—but you won't have the comforts of our expert advice.

From Dr. Golding's office, we were diverted back to the lobby. A few minutes later a personable young male orderly, in a uniform reminiscent of a hotel bellboy, entered with a wheelchair, and I—who had walked all over until now—rode the last mile in wretched dejection. I always feel embarrassed when they do this. I try to hide by squeezing down into my seat, but it doesn't help. It only makes you more conspicuous. As you pass people in the halls, they all glance at you with a knowing smile. "Amateur!" They say. You can see it all over their face. They can spot us every time.

They did the same thing in Akron. I had driven the car all day and gone to meetings. I had walked at the mall. I had driven to the doctor's and back to my home. I had walked into admitting, standing fully erect. But the moment I signed those admitting forms, they did it to me. Waiting in the wings was a nurse with one of those things! The hospitals in Akron are, in this respect, a step ahead of the clinic in capturing male patients, because they always send their prettiest girls to do the job; no matter how much you wish it otherwise, it's pretty hard to refuse to sit in that chair. Like the Lorelei on the Rhine and the nymphs of Greece, women have ruled males much longer than history has recorded, or than we care to admit.

7

PREPARING
FOR
OPERATION

The orderly who wheeled me onto the elevator and up to my room was a black with a charming personality. I poured out my soul to him, and he joked and laughed with me until we reached the room. He was a good choice for the job.

The room was semiprivate and the bed near the window was occupied. The occupant was an old-timer who was surrounded by his middle-aged children and their spouses. They flashed me a friendly smile as I rolled in, but I glared back. This wasn't the private room I had ordered, I snorted to myself. Admitting had assured me that no private rooms were available, but I figured by now they could have found one. I reached over and pulled the drape around my bed, so I could get into my hospital gown, with the sexy split in the back. But as soon as the drape cut the room in two, my neighbor's daughter whipped it open so she could talk.

My wife and she struck up a lively chatter while I tried to close the drape once more to regain my privacy. But she held on to the drape, and I could budge it only a couple of feet. I finally gave up with a glare at my wife and changed as privately as I could underneath my gown. I felt like I had the lead role in an R-rated movie.

These people turned out to be pleasant enough, once you got past being overwhelmed by a roomful of gossips; by the time the old-timer went for his operation the next day, I found myself wishing him well. The family even stayed for an hour or two to chat with me. Like those who practice a life of crime, heart patients and their relatives have much to pull them into a common orbit. Everyone wants to learn of your problems and to be reassured by any kind of straw they can hang on to. Once a patient leaves this room, that's the last mile. The family is as alone and frightened as the patient. These people came from Lansing, and Cleveland was new to them, so they felt even more lonely. The old fellow went bravely. He smiled a little bit, but his face was tight, and I could see he was frightened, but too proud to admit it—like James Cagney on his way to the electric chair, I thought. That was a good movie, by the way. I saw it again recently, and Cagney started screaming in the end. This guy never did. Maybe he should have had the part.

This fellow almost had a heart attack the night I arrived. He had warned me several times that evening about a mad orderly that the hospital used for shaving its patients. All patients are shaved before they go into surgery, because hair is full of bacteria. But what a shave! They strip you completely and spread you out on your bed with a sheet of icy plastic stretched under you. Then they soak you down and lather you up. The orderly starts at your chin (you get to keep the hair on your head and your day's growth of face whiskers), and he whips off every hair you own between the chin and the shin, front and back. Nothing stays. When you look at your body afterwards, it looks like a plucked chicken hung out to dry. No wonder home is such a pleasant place to be, when you think of all the tricks played on the human race by our fellow humans.

These orderlies work so fast, whipping that razor back and forth (I think they are paid on piecework basis, so much per head) that you scarcely expect to have any skin left when they get through. That was the problem. My neighbor did lose a number of chunks, here and there.

Naturally, after the shave, you take a shower using an iodized soap wash, to clean and disinfect yourself. When he did this, my roommate's body stung so badly he had an angina attack. Then he had trouble sleeping. He got up several times that night and complained. I almost shouted at him to keep his light off so I could get some sleep, but I didn't want that on my conscience at such a critical moment.

I thought to myself at the time, They didn't do this to James Cagney. When his time came, they gave him a full meal.

By the time my turn came, I was so frightened that I kept hoping the barber would forget to show up. If that happened, I figured they'd have to take me into surgery with all my hair on.

To protect myself, in any event, I proceeded from the next morning on to plead with everyone I saw not to let that orderly (barber) in my room. Even my surgeon was not exempt.

Dr. Golding stopped in to see me on the afternoon before my operation. He came to discuss the operation and reconfirm my schedule, but I wanted instead to talk about the razorwielder, whom I feared much more. The orderly was due that night, and the operation was not until the next morning. And I wanted to take them in order, one at a time.

Dr. Golding must have wondered about the strange priorities of a patient about to have his heart tampered with who was more worried about a shave. He patiently promised to place me under his protection.

When he left, I figured he probably shook his head in disbelief and forgot about it, but I soon learned he was true to his word.

From then on every nurse that entered my room commented on it sympathetically, and I soon became embarrassed at my popularity as the number one chicken.

When the orderly did appear, it was a different person, a young black man who was studying in college and did this kind of work in the evenings to make some money. When he entered the room, Beethoven was on the radio, and his first comment was that he liked Beethoven. This set the stage, and from then on my whole attitude improved. This *Barbiera di Seviglia* of mine whipped his razor about with the speed of a rapier, and it was a marvel to behold and a terror to endure. I shivered from the cold, but when he was done, I was unscathed. He had left the complete operation to Dr. Golding. My fears had been for naught. Unlike the other barber, he was resigned to the fact that he was not a practicing surgeon, only an orderly! But at that he was good.

My roommate who had gone before me had not only suffered from the preoperative tortures of an unskilled barber but had also found himself the victim of a separate cruel turn of fate. On the morning of his operation, he was aroused at 6 A.M. by a nurse and told to prepare himself. His family came on board, and all the lights in the room were flung on. I pretended to sleep, but someone in the entourage spotted my one eye popping open and immediately pounced on me. I could not even pretend to sleep.

When the poor guy was ready to be wheeled down the

hall, nothing happened. They never came for him. Time dragged on, and he was notified that an emergency had arisen and his operation would be delayed.

The delay dragged on until 2 P.M. He never got to eat all day; the family fidgeted, and the strain began to show on their faces. Finally, the men in the white coats came for him with a mattressed chariot—a bed on wheels instead of a wheelchair. As he rode off, I hated to see him go. The room suddenly became quiet and lonely. He survived the operation, I learned several days later, and did very well.

Just a few minutes after he left my room, they wheeled in another patient. The nurse's aide had hardly had time to change the sheets. This new roommate had already been through the operation and was transferred to my room for a final stay prior to shipping out for home.

He was the law director of a small town in northern Ohio. It was an appointive post, apparently subject to approval and recall by the town council. He had hardly reached my room when his phone rang: a friend of his calling to tell him that a plot was afoot to replace him. His enemies had apparently seized the opportunity of his absence to mount a coup. They had waited too long, however, because he was not as helpless as his enemies had hoped. They should have nailed him the day of the operation, but fate was working for him.

As soon as he learned of the abortive plot, he called all his supporters and associates and mounted a counterattack. He was on that phone, either calling or being called, for several hours. Apparently the council was meeting that evening to make the decision. Since all the calls were long-distance, his phone bill that day must have exceeded his room bill, which was a sizable accomplishment for a sick man.

Finally the calls stopped, and the room was silent for an hour or so. He and I talked. He seemed to be thoroughly enjoying himself. There was no sign of weariness. His voice was strong and effective during the whole period.

I learned that he had had the job for eighteen years. He obviously knew his way around. This may not have been his first experience of this type.

Finally the phone rang again, and he was informed that he had won. Once more he began a series of calls to thank all his supporters. He was on the phone until long after I had gone to sleep. I was tired and he was still going strong. The miracle of healing had certainly blessed him. I hoped to do as well.

During the next day he had no visitors, and I never did find out if he was married. His home was about three hours' drive, and with all his phone calls he may have superseded the need for personal visits, because he kept the phone as busy the second day as he did the first night. Between calls, we talked, or he talked to the nurses.

I found out that prior to being evacuated to my room, he had spent five days in unit 7Q. There he had gotten to know the nurses. From my own personal experiences, it appeared that he must have awakened from his operation chatting with the staff. His popularity was such that three of the nurses from the seventh floor came to visit him at his new room. I never had achieved such heights of popularity. In fact, when I would walk down the halls after my operation and meet the nurses, they didn't even know me.

He was generous, however, in his friendships. When nurse friends came to our room to visit him, he introduced them to me as well and told them I was to be their next boarder. They were delighted, they said, and told me to request unit 7Q for my postoperative recovery. That's the place where the staff and patients all got together every evening for a cocktail hour, they told me suggestively. Naturally, I rose to the bait and resolved not to forget about unit 7Q. No man is ever so sick that he passes up the chance to be indulged during his recovery. In fact, the two are synonymous, I believed, and I was glad to see that the clinic agreed.

Visualizing dancing girls and evenings of debauchery, in my semidemented state, I was pleased with my change in fortune. After all, my companion was the same age as I, and here were three pretty nurses visiting him. So I asked them how I could arrange my schedule to end up in 7Q. "Tell the nurse on the morning of your operation," they advised me, "and she will write a note on your arm, 'Return to 7Q.'" The prospects of being so labeled struck me as incongruous. Somewhat like a slab of bacon, I saw myself (still unconscious) being routed through the building, my arm being checked at

each station. After thirty years of telling others how to schedule production and how to move material from operation to
operation, I had now become the material and my arm was the
move ticket. It fitted the classic production situation completely: Seventeen operations a day were being done at the
clinic; a doctor at my daughter's hospital would soon be an-
nouncing his thousandth operation and would celebrate its
anniversary; there were now 100,000 cases of this type each
year in the United States alone.

Having passed through its infancy with an unsurpassed
record for improvement and survival, the operation now was
creating less interest than a common cold. The only ones who
seemed to care anymore, I learned later, were the patient, the
family, and the hospital. For the others, the operation had lost
its bite. It was no longer party conversation. To mention it in a
crowd, where it once created a hushed silence like you were
an E.F. Hutton broker, they now looked at you like you were
born without manners. That's the price you pay for a record of
safety. You must choose your operations carefully and in a
timely manner if you are to get full mileage from them. In this
respect, my first operation was far more exciting. Second
operations still have some novelty value, but it's not the same
as it used to be. Who pays attention to the current generation
of astronauts, our unsung heroes?

These ideas never really passed through my head at the
time, but they do now. Today, when I see my friends, they talk
about the weather. They have thirty other friends with bypasses and have one of their own scheduled.

You saw that I had checked in a few days early at the clinic
to give them time to check me out and get me educated. But
my political roommate followed a different pattern. He entered the hospital the day of his operation. The clinic was trying a
new program out on him to see if total hospital time could be
reduced safely. In his case, he got the same tests and training I
did, but as an outpatient. Even the morning of the operation,
he drove to the clinic from home, arrived early, and was
shaved. From there he went directly onto the table and into
the operation. His recovery, as you saw, was remarkable. In
fact, he went home the day I had my operation. (He called

back a couple of days later to see how I was doing—and I can't even vote for him. Does this mean he was really a nice guy after all?)

Most people are given the more formal treatment, like I got. If you are one of them, you arrive the night before and are checked out by several staff doctors from cardiology.

The next day you are sent to spirometry, where you breathe into a special machine. You take a deep breath and blow out as hard as you can. This is done to test your lung capacity. You get a chest x-ray and an ECG. You again meet Dr. Golding and Dr. Sheldon. Dr. Sheldon was my cardiologist while at the clinic. He visited me each day during my stay there, and for as little time as we had to get to know each other, I was impressed with his ability and manner. He was a particularly warm individual and extremely capable. He was chairman of the department. I was very pleased with Dr. Ormond's choice to represent him while I was at the clinic. As you have seen, I had been very disturbed by the abrupt disruption involved in severing my contacts in Akron and the prospects of beginning completely anew in Cleveland. I should not have been. The people at the clinic, especially Dr. Sheldon, were absolutely great to work with. I would have no hesitation to go back to the clinic if I could repeat my experiences. Because the people in a facility are a reflection of the leaders, the warmth of the clinic in dealing with total strangers (who form the bulk of its patients) speaks highly of the personal qualities of Dr. Sheldon. As you will see in my later notes, I have continued my treatment under Dr. Ormond, because I respect him very highly—and am no longer mad at him. But I am also grateful now to have a second line of communication established. I have always believed in getting two viewpoints, one to confirm the other. This makes good sense in operations as serious as this. But two viewpoints are not easy to obtain in times of emergency, unless they have been previously established. When an emergency arises under most circumstances, you are usually forced to depend entirely upon the wisdom and your judgment of the competence of the one man who says you must commit your life to him. Fortunately, for me, Dr. Ormond was a dedicated man of great personal integrity and skill in his profession, and my earlier experiences with him have all been corroborated by later observations.

Today, the Cleveland Clinic now represents a second, corroborative force that eases the mind of the many doubts that creep in, both before and even years after the operation. Because of the many nasty rumors that abound about the medical profession in the news and the public's mind, there are always little doubts that nag you as to whether the operation was really necessary. Not often, but sometimes, you wonder if, just maybe, you could have done as well by simply taking medicine and being more careful. These doubts are silly, as you've seen, but they surfaced in the past; and as my health and general well-being improve with the passage of time, since my second operation, I suspect that they will arise again.

For one thing, our experiences of the past tell us, in Pavlovian manner, that illnesses come to an end with the passage of time. Time cures illness. When we get a cold or the flu, for example, no matter how sick we are, we soon feel better. I suspect that this syndrome stays with us in life so that, following the operation, when we feel healthy and energetic again and the pains are almost completely forgotten, we relegate our heart problems in our mind to the status of a bad cold. We wonder to ourselves if time would not have been the great healer here as well.

As I have said, the news media don't help in this respect; quite the contrary, they plant doubts in the public's mind, long before an individual is ever called upon to make such an important decision.

The doctors at the clinic are a particularly dedicated lot. They serve at a fixed salary that is ample but not excessive. They are not permitted to engage in private practice. As a result, they are much like college professors, in the European style, serving with great prestige and dedication. Hence, although the clinic supports a number of research activities, the costs at the clinic are comparable to those in Akron and other cities.

The process of testing and interviewing goes on all day. A battery of lab tests is made: Blood is drawn for analysis.

Your pulse is checked regularly. Your blood pressure is recorded.

At 3 P.M. you are sent to a breathing class, under the direction of a respiratory therapist, who in my case was a male nurse. Here you learn the importance of breathing deeply and coughing to clear the lungs. During the operation and the postoperative period, the lungs tend to collect fluids that must be expunged. or else you will contract pneumonia. Each person in the class is given a funny plastic tube with a hose and mouthpiece attached. Inside the tube is a little ball that rises to the top as you inhale. You are asked to inhale and raise the ball to the top, and keep holding the ball up, while you time yourself. Your best time is recorded. Even before the operation, some patients can only keep the ball in the air for a couple of seconds. Others can do it for fifteen seconds or longer.

After leaving the class, you are given the device to take to your room and told to practice with it. It will be used after the operation, when you awaken. You will use it every two hours, to force yourself to breath deeply. After every two or three breaths on the machine, you are supposed to cough as deeply as possible, sitting upright on the bed, holding your chest with a pillow. A therapist stands by to help you expel the fluids, pounding on your back while you cough.

Because the open heart operation involves laying your ribs wide open like a chicken, the closing procedure involves wiring the ribs together to hold them in place. Hence, your first reaction on waking up is that coughing is going to blow your chest wide open. It's hard, therefore, to convince yourself that coughing is beneficial. The pillow held tightly to your chest helps, because psychologically you think it keeps you together. It does help reduce the pain, but the pain is less of a problem than the fear of undoing yourself.

At 4 P.M. you go to another class, this time with your spouse or some other member of the family. Here you learn some of the details of what's going to happen to you during the next few days. Your family is told how they can get up-to-date messages on your progress, where to wait during the operation, and whom to see. Families are given a number to call if they go home and instructions on leaving a number where they can be reached. The briefing is thorough and is followed by a period of questions and answers.

Both Akron City and the Cleveland Clinic Hospital give dietary classes for heart patients. These classes covered foods that were low in salt, the use of salt substitutes, avoiding animal fats, and the questions of cholesterol that were on everyone's lips. In both classes, the views on cholesterol were identical. Cholesterol is less dogmatically condemned than it was at the time of my first operation. Doctors apparently sit on both sides of the question, so that the dietitian discusses the latest state of the art but sets forth no absolute restrictions.

Despite the busy schedule, I found time to visit a close friend from Akron. He was a patient on the floor below mine and had been admitted eight weeks earlier for a metal knee insert. While there, he ran into a series of heart-breaking setbacks, including a gallbladder operation and an infection in the knee that finally forced the doctors to remove the knee joint and fuse the bones together. His mental outlook had deteriorated badly. He was released only the day before me, and his experiences had been so traumatic that he openly resented my good fortune and quick recovery. This resentment passed when he got home, and we may be closer friends now than ever, since we have more in common to share together.

It is four months later as I write this. Within three weeks of my operation I was driving my car, and in two months I was working full-time at my job. He is still not back to work full-time. His leg is still in a cast, and he has more to come. He works only one or two hours a day.

We frequently do not know how lucky we are. It is difficult to appreciate how far the profession has come in treating the most critical of all body organs. Once heart patients had no future.

The night before the operation you receive your regular meal in your room. Then you are shaved, as we discussed earlier, and about 10 A.M. you are given a sleeping pill. Quite contrary to the joke everyone tells about hospitals, no one ever woke me up to give me a sleeping pill—in either hospital. This may be because I tended to do my sleeping at night rather than night and day, as many patients do.

In my case, the night before the operation it had begun

snowing, and the wind was blowing badly. Being almost Christmas, it got dark early, so I encouraged my wife to leave early. The bad weather was a threat because she would have to leave home quite early the next morning to be at the hospital by 6 A.M. My operation was scheduled for 7.

This was one of the saddest moments of my life, when she left. It was Christmas everywhere: on TV, on the radio, and in the decorated halls. I truly hated to be alone that evening. A friendly law director and a hospital room could not take the place of my home and my family on a night like this. I had to choke back the tears.

When the barber came, about 10 P.M., the distraction wasn't welcome, but it occupied my mind and gave me a fresh start.

After my shower, I took a sleeping pill and fell soundly asleep. I never woke up again until they turned the lights on and awakened me. My wife, my youngest daughter, Jacqueline, and her husband Mark entered the room a few minutes later. The big moment was at hand. It was December 18.

THE RIDE DOWN THE CORRIDOR

Getting Close to God

December 18! I was still sitting on the bed, rubbing sleep from my eyes, when I saw my family. I don't recall the next thirty minutes in detail. I went to the bathroom, washed my face, and scrubbed my teeth. The few possessions I had—my watch, my slippers, my pajama bottoms—I gave to my wife to take home. Things seem to have moved rapidly, because hospital attendants arrived with a bed on wheels. I crawled on top and slid under a sheet, and the cart was pushed into the corridor. My family followed alongside. I remember my wife's strained face. She looked worried. I smiled at her. Because I was on my back, the overhead lights in the hall hurt my eyes as they glided by. They reminded me of a TV program I saw once in which the camera took just such a view of those overhead lights. It must have been a Ben Casey or Dr. Kildare movie. I thought of this as we moved down the hall. The cart stopped at the induction room. At the door, I kissed my wife and daughter. Then, while they trudged to the family lounge, I was wheeled into the room to be prepared for the operation.

These times are worse for the family than the patient. By now the patient has made peace with himself. He has accepted his fate. There was no desire on my part to jump off the cart and tell everyone I had changed my mind. In fact, such a thought never crossed my mind. That phase of my life had passed during my stay at home. A calm had settled upon me, and I am not sure that there were any signs of nervousness. In discussions with Ginny since the operation, she has never mentioned any, although she did say I was very fidgety at the first operation.

This is a natural condition. Most people feel nervous before important events. Nervousness or anxiety before an operation is as normal as it is for athletes before an important game. It is usually alleviated by discussions with your doctor and understanding the reasons for the operation. Mild medication, which is usually given an hour before the operation to produce drowsiness, also helps.

Naturally, my second operation had the benefit of prior experience, but there were other changes involved. This transition can be seen in the following incident.

The night before my first operation, a man entered my room. He introduced himself as Reverend David Burnham. I knew who he was by name, if not by face. My wife and brother-in-law had gone to his church for years. They liked him, as did a large section of the city of Akron. He had one of the largest congregations in the area. I had never been impressed. He was a fundamentalist. He shouted at times, which irritated me. He spoke too long, which also irritated me. I liked teachers, not preachers, and he was too much of the latter. I didn't even like the building he was in. It was a large, modern structure that was more like an auditorium than a cathedral. It was clean and neat, which gave the operation good points for efficiency.

When he introduced himself, I told him I wasn't about to become a hypocrite at this late juncture in life and that I didn't need his help. He was startled, and I could see the shock in his face as he walked to the door and turned back to see if I had had a change of heart.

I suspected the hand of my brother-in-law in this. With a congregation of over 10,000 members, the minister had little reason to single me out from his nonmembership to pay a visit. It was a clear case of prior plotting. I appreciated his dedication to duty and generosity with his personal time, but not his mission. I needed no Bible-toting sycophant urging me to recant and confess sins I had not committed and felt no remorse over.

My only remorse was that I had not been more tactful; I wasn't particularly concerned with my relationship with God. I felt God knew me well enough to need no intermediary.

Because death, nearness to death, and religious awe are intertwined in the human mind, you would expect that all people who come close to death also come close to God. That they welcome preachers and holy men. But at least in my case, I felt uneasy in his presence and resentful for his impudent intrusion.

Seeking religious solace at times like these may be true for many, but it does not square with my own experiences, which appear to run upstream, counter to the common pattern. God and I have always been on a teeter-totter. Sometimes He's allowed in my life; other times I've kept Him out.

There have been large segments of my life in which I have hardly been aware of a dependency, or an acknowledgment of His existence. I am even embarrassed to suggest such an idea, now, on paper.

I went through three and a half years in the Navy, of which half was in the war zones in the Atlantic and Pacific. I've seen bombings, strafings, kamikazis, planes shot down, and ships gutted, but seldom felt any interest in church or need for God. And yet in the back of my mind, He must have been there. An incident toward the end of the war makes me think this. It was the announced bombing of Japan with the atom bomb. I found it so incredulous that man could invent such a thing that my first reaction, spoken out loud, was, "God would not permit such a bomb."

Obviously—I have since learned—God doesn't place limits on the human race. Mankind is supposed to govern itself, rightly or wrongly. We can go as far as we want, because that is how we progress. No child learns without making mistakes. Some are costly but unavoidable. It is more costly still for the human race, however, to stop progress in the name of safety and fear for the future. Caution may be prudent, but never should we discourage exploration and advancement.

This was about as close as I got to God until I got married. And then I remember that I was again overwhelmed with a sense of beauty and piety.

Following college, and a few years of working for others, I started my own management consulting business. It went very well, and the better it went, the less interest I showed in God, the less important He became. My success came from my abilities and my decisions.

It didn't come from my church attendance. In fact, church attendance declined with time or held steady at one or two services a year: Christmas and Easter. I only went to hear the music. I had an almost perfect record of attendance, on this basis, until the church began to put more stress on modern forms of music. Being fundamentalist in its preachings, it maintained one foot in the past and one in the future by appealing to the youth of America, who enjoyed rock over Bach. This was all right for them, but it completed my exodus from the church.

Having lost my last contact, I gave up the ghost and stayed home. Not even the heart operation shook my feelings. God was available to me through my own devices, and I felt compelled to call upon Him rarely. If I needed Him, He was there. Much of the time, I wasn't sure He even existed. In my colder, more sober moments I could see no reason why He should exist.

I still have fleeting fits of these feelings at times. Some doubts creep in, in my more independent moments, but they are quickly crowded out today by other experiences. As a result, I feel that I've had a change of heart. I've gotten more religious.

I'm not a Bible-toting, lapel-grabbing zealot, mind you, like some I've known that drive you for cover. Until this book, I've been a closet type of believer in religion and its benefits. I'm still not sure I'd welcome any preacher coming around to pray over me. He can save that till I'm dead, if at all.

No doubt the heart operation played a role in this transition, this softening of my position, but it was a delayed role. If I had died on the operating table, it might have been too late for me. My amends had not been made. That did not come until later. Perhaps it was a stubborn streak, or a wish not to be a hypocrite even before God. At any rate, what seems to have changed my outlook was a streak of bad luck in business. The god of greed that had served so well lost his power to attract me.

As a consultant to management, my job was to advise, and in this respect I had established a successful, well-respected business. But other challenges developed, and I found myself directly involved in the excitement of running operations themselves. I became a doer as well as a teacher. I had had several early successes turning businesses around for clients, making losers profitable. So I decided I could make more money and have more fun by investing funds of my own in these firms and reaping the overall rewards. This worked well. My first efforts were very successful, and I moved quickly to expand into several companies at once. By the time of my first operation, I was involved in turning three firms around simultaneously, one of them in Texas and the other two in the Midwest.

In addition, I owned and operated a 66,000-acre ranch in Utah, running 500 head of cattle.

All of these operations required constant attention and travel. In addition, they required financing to support them until they could support themselves. Most of my time was spent negotiating with creditors, to maintain the flow of materials, and in dealing with banks. Then, two weeks before my first visit to the hospital, a chink fell out of place when the ranch manager left to take a job with an oil company in Saudi Arabia.

My attention span and energy were diverted by the health problems over the next few months, and the whole house of cards began to tremble. Large sections began to collapse, and my cash flow became increasingly negative. Under prior health conditions, I would have thrown myself into the problem with energy and might have reversed the trend. But I lacked the physical stamina and spiritual strength called for. From the moment of the operation, I had resolved to simplify my business affairs rather than saddle my family with them. But as fast as I attempted to reorganize one area, other problems developed, so that I spent my time putting out fires instead of solving problems. From the day I got out of the hospital, I was constantly on the phone. As conditions worsened, I became despondent and frightened.

As my world collasped around me I feared for my ability to support my family. I still had no idea how much I could depend upon my health, which seemed to be fragile. I found myself traveling constantly and dreading to leave home.

The heart problem had frightened me more than I cared to admit, and I lacked the inner fortitude needed to face the situation. (As it turned out, I regained my physical stamina— at least equal to that of much earlier—as soon as my financial problems were washed away. But while the fears of financial disaster plagued me, I lived in constant terror of the future, and I was unable to operate at full capacity.)

It was during this period that I began to pray with concentrated effort and to beg for help. I realized now that if I was to come to grips with my situation, I needed help from outside of myself. I surely wasn't getting much help from within.

As my financial problems unraveled, I regained my confidence and my energy. I rebuilt my consulting business. My income went from minus to plus. It gradually reached its former levels. My energy and output multiplied. I learned to function in a more effective, more leisurely manner, without all the close timing and pressures. Then, the year before my second operation, my output became prodigious. I wrote two books on management and at the same time maintained an active consulting business. One book was published in June, and the other arrived in the mail on the very day before I entered the clinic.

This renewal of my heart condition was not caused, in my opinion, by my workload. I never let it get heavy or burdensome; I watched my pace carefully. I spent a great deal of time with the family. Rather, I think it was a product of the enormous pressures I had been under during those intervening years prior to getting my affairs straightened out. We read how people commit suicide when they are in financial distress. The Great Depression ruined many men financially who took their own lives. I wonder if we don't indirectly do this same thing with our health. Do people indirectly try to commit suicide, in an honorable way, by bringing on serious health problems? What about the first heart problem? Was it preceded by a similar type of condition? A similar death wish?

I believe it was. As I look back, my finances had taken a bad swing about two years before the first problem. The conditions had been different and I had straightened them out successfully, reaching new heights in accumulation. But the stress and fears had been there. I had been frightened, but my health had been good, and I could depend on myself in the long run. It wasn't until both problems, money and health, faced me that I realized my dependence on something bigger than myself. If I was broken down both financially and physically, my prospects for the future were terrifying.

Have others had experiences such as these? Are there, in other words, conditions that precede the operation which are analogous to my own? To answer these questions I got on the phone and arranged luncheon meetings with several friends to see what might have triggered their own experiences.

Robert L. King, a highly successful realtor from Wellington, was forty-five when he had his operation. About a year to eighteen months earlier he had gone through the trauma of a divorce. He had three children and a beautiful home that he had built on a large farm a few years before, so the impact of these recent events on his life was understandably serious. Bob was a close family man, and after the final separation, two of the children (who were in high school) made their home with him.

Another close friend became deeply involved with another woman. He also had children and a well-established professional life. As his involvement became deeper, he was forced to choose between his family and his girlfriend.

As he tells it, his wife never knew of his affair with the other woman, or at least she wisely kept silent and bore her pain within.

His girlfriend pressured him to break with his wife, and for months he agonized over the decision. He loved the girl very much, but he also loved his wife and couldn't hurt his family. In the end, he chose his family, but the experience culminated in a heart attack about a year later.

From a close associate I heard about another case involving a man who was a partner with his brother in a manufacturing plant. The firm reached a sales level in excess of $10 million. He became an active playboy, joining numerous elite country clubs. He apparently suffered a minor heart attack at about this time and began to suffer from angina. He went through open heart surgery, and shortly after that his business failed completely, ending in bankruptcy. This example is interesting because of another twist involved: This man suffered a severe personality change.

None of my own acquaintances became involved in significant changes in personality. They were the same persons after the operation as before, except that all of them seemed to be less driven afterwards. They seemed to have mellowed. All were entrepreneurs, and all had successful records and high incomes. After the operation there was a visible slacking off in drive, but not necessarily a reduction in success, although there was frequently a bad stumble, suggesting that these people were living with very little slack in the line. As one of them said to me, "I don't get upset with people anymore, and things just seem to happen anyway. I'm more understanding now, and I think I do a better job than I did before, when I tried to push people to get things done. I've always been able to motivate people but have never been happy with their level of accomplishment."

The change in personality, on the other hand, that took place in the individual described by my friend was radical in character and certainly unpredictable. This man and his lawyer had grown up together. They were close friends. The attorney sat on his board and served both as the company attorney and as his personal lawyer. As the man's company collapsed, the attorney's fees became quite substantial. The heart patient abandoned the attorney, switched to a new lawyer, and filed for personal bankruptcy, wiping out the debt he owed his former friend. In addition to alienating himself from the lawyer, this man no longer talks to his brother. He has virtually isolated himself from his past. He seems to be a man who is lost and frightened and has nothing to hang on to. Open heart patients sometimes suffer a stroke. Perhaps this happened.

One final example is provided by a man I met at the clinic on one of my visits to the postoperative ward. This man had been operated on only four days before I interviewed him. He was only forty-seven and was surprisingly strong. His voice was firm, and he moved about with considerable ease. He was teaching school when he had his attack. He thought it was the flu. He lost his balance and hit the blackboard. He did not see a doctor until three days later. (This seems to be a common experience. Many people with heart problems think it's the flu or a gallbladder attack or something else. They seldom think it's their heart. Maybe this is a form of escape mechanism.)

Prior to becoming a teacher, he had been a builder. He had gone into teaching to obtain more security and get away from the pressures.

A year and a half before his operation, his father, to whom he had been very close, died. At the same time, he became involved in an experience in which he was threatened with the loss of a large investment. He had placed a substantial down payment on a home and later found out that the seller owed more on the house than it was worth. He should have placed the money in escrow, but for some reason he gave it directly to the seller. Getting his money back involved legal problems and a long, difficult period of time, with great stress.

This man told me he had a violent temper and that he would get so mad, when he was a builder, that he would swing at the house or throw his tools around. He also worked two jobs for many years, showing both the drive and cooped-up energy that we saw in the other examples.

All of these men seemed to depend on themselves for their results so that when things went wrong, they felt the failures deeply within themselves. In other words, they tended to be loners. They had not developed the habit of depending upon others when they needed help.

These few examples would hardly carry much weight in a court of law, but here again I have been fortunate in coming across an actual report on the subject by an authority far more reliable than I. The report was given by Dr. Harvey Brenner, a professor at Johns Hopkins University, to the Joint Economic Committee of Congress in the fall of 1980. Professor Brenner estimates that with each increase in unemployment of one percentage point during a recession, there will be about 37,000 deaths over the period of the next six years. Of these, more than 20,000 will die of cardiovascular problems caused by *stress and poor diet*. Some of these are suicides, but others are spread out over a six-year period following the increase in unemployment.

We cannot interview these unfortunate souls, of course, to find out how lonely they must have felt, or how dejected. We can only sense their problem.

In my own case, as I began to suspect that there was something out there besides me, my mental and physical attitudes improved. My confidence returned, and my fortunes improved. This time I resolved not to go it alone but to stick with all the help I could get. Independence had been great—until I found myself all alone in the world. But I found that the spiritual help was a nice crutch to lean on. Furthermore, it didn't cramp my style too greatly. I could do much as I had before, but I now had a conscience to give my decisions validity and to guide me. Living with this condition imposed on my freedom turned out to be no serious handicap to my hopes for the future. In fact, it probably helped. I'm not where I once was financially. I haven't recovered everything. But I'm not sure it really makes any difference. It's not that important.

Today, I appreciate my family and my friends so much

more. My wife and I are closer to our children, including the married ones, than we ever were before. As a group, we do many things together. We enjoy each other's company. Two of my children work for me part-time. My daughter Kathleen, for example, typed this, as she did my other books. Ten years before, we had tried the same arrangement, and it hadn't worked at all. It had only resulted in bitterness and criticism.

Having found a better way to move forward in life, I resolved to stick with it, once my fortunes changed. In the depths of despair, it's easy to seek out God. But to stick with Him, to retain your relationship when things go right, is less easy. When He's not needed for moral support, He's forgotten or discarded. Then He's hard to pick back up later, because you're out of practice. Your "hot line" to God has gotten rusty and full of static from disuse. You may not be able to get through at all, if you've overplayed your hand.

I was lucky, I felt, so I decided to stick with my new routine. Sure, I waver every once in a while, but I usually get reinforcements along the way that keep me on the track.

What happened, of course, is that my state of mind was better prepared for the second operation than the first. Sure, I resented it as an imposition on my life; I hated the idea of being totally dependent for long periods; I dreaded the few days surrounding the operation because of the pain and discomfort; I dreaded the uncertainty of the future. After all, it offered no guarantees. I could be a permanent invalid or worse, and I could not provide my wife with a secure financial future. We had just regained our financial feet, and now we faced extremely heavy medical expenses only partly covered by medical insurance.

So I prayed and kept on praying.

In some respects I looked forward to the prospect of dying—not as an escape from the past but as a flight into the future. To be sure, there had been a lot of problems here on earth, as you've seen. My life insurance was in good shape, with the additional amounts I had been lucky enough to get. Hence, my family was in better shape, by far, with me dead than alive, especially if I ended up as an invalid.

But there was another factor involved as well. My philosophical nature and background in college had always piqued my curiosity. Why was the earth created? How was it created?

What is the purpose of man on earth? Why are we here? How does life function beyond the veil? Like the majority of the people here on earth, my wife had never been bothered by these wonderings. She was a perfect mother who never questioned church or dogma. She dutifully attended church and listened to every word the preacher said, as if it had been spoken by God Himself. By contrast, I questioned everything he said and shuddered at his dogmatic narrow-mindedness. I wanted to see for myself, to get the answers firsthand, but she was happy to have the thing handed to her on a platter. Hence, I saw this operation as an opportunity to step across the line into the hereafter with no pain or suffering. I'm no different than many others: Death isn't the frightening prospect. It's not death we fear but getting it over with: the long period of suffering and human decay that eventually closes the door on life.

As a result of these kinds of thoughts, my trip to the operating room was not nearly as frightening as it could have been. In some respects I was excited over the prospects of a new experience, above and beyond the present world. I wanted to see what lay beyond, what the answers were to questions that the mind could only surmise. Of all those old philosophers of Greece, Germany, and England, had any been right?

It should come as no surprise to you, then, that the first few days of my recovery, I felt a sad sense of having been cheated. This pervaded my psyche for days. After fifty-seven years of questioning all religions and searching for answers, I had thought them about to be known. Instead, I was back where I started. I would have to wait again before I learned the truth. How long would this third wait be? Would the final end be painless or sudden? Only God knows. I was back where I had started.

Of course I'm glad to be alive and to be doing so well. As time has passed, I've become more than happy with my fate. I doubt if I would change it if I had a chance. But you are entitled to the truth, as it happened; and that is what I have given you.

I go to church regularly now, hoping to fill some of the gaps and improve my communication with the Almighty. I'm still not a perfectly good churchgoer. Many of the doubts and problems I mentioned earlier still consume my questioning soul. I still study the other religions to see if they can tell me something.

I still don't usually enjoy preaching, but I keep hoping a bolt of lightning will hit. I still have my own private little church service, which I need for myself. I encourage the family to attend church because I would be eternally grateful to need no more than my wife seeks from religion.

As I compare the first and second episodes of my life, I can see enormous advantages to finding a meaningful relationship with God. It took me many years and enormous stresses, but the last couple of years have been some of my best. You may question my precocity as a rank amateur in this field, but I feel that we who have been closest to death speak with a special authority not given to those others.

To conclude this chapter, I have asked Dr. Ormond and the Reverend David Burnham to give you their thoughts on the relationship between medicine and God. Dr. Ormond is a member of Dr. Burnham's church, the same church I attend. We all met under completely different circumstances. When I first met Dr. Ormond, I had been unaware of his affiliation with Dr. Burnham's church. We ran into each other, as it happened, leaving church one Sunday. His feelings on religion and medicine are of immense significance. I hope you will feel the same.

Dr. Burnham is here to give you a professional cleric's view of God and serious heart problems. His views have obviously influenced me, even though I have been coming to them slowly and with great resistance.

A DOCTOR LOOKS AT RELIGION
Alexander P. Ormond, Jr.,M.D.
Cardiologist, Akron City Hospital

In my practice of medicine I find that many patients have a spiritual hunger that can be satisfied only by abiding faith in Jesus Christ as their Savior. This hunger is manifested in patients who have all forms of medical problems, but it is especially evident in patients who are facing serious heart problems and who are about to undergo heart surgery. The results of modern-day heart surgery are improving all the time, and the risks are relatively low, but the patients are still apprehensive and need to be able to turn to God for solace in their time of crisis. I believe that patients in these situations want to know that if they turn to God as true believers, their prayers are heard and answered and that if something should go awry with the surgery, they can look forward to spending eternity in heaven. If patients have this knowledge prior to surgery and have become true believers, it is very easy to counsel them, for they have a peace that is not present in those who have no faith. I advise patients that they need to be in prayer so that they can be at peace with themselves and have comfort in going to sleep and knowing that their destiny is in God's hands. If patients don't have this peace, then I, as a physician, should do everything to try to provide them with the secure knowledge of where their destiny lies. Some patients reject this advice, and I can only pray that they wake up after surgery, for if they don't, they will be lost forever.

After observing hundreds of patients who are facing heart surgery, it's clear that those who are spiritually secure are more comfortable in placing themselves in the position of possibly not surviving the surgery. They have a greater peace about them and are much less agitated before, and after, surgery. If the surgery should be unsuccessful, as it occasionally is, the patients are more likely to be able to accept this. Spiritual peace is a tremendous advantage for coping with everyday living and also for coping with crises that arise when your health fails.

These comments by Dr. Ormond, though very short, are beautifully stated. Perhaps in analogy, some of the most beautiful music ever written—Schubert's Serenade, *La Golondrina*, "Silent Night"—was also short. Simplicity and grace of style are gifts we can all enjoy.

The closing of this chapter has been reserved for Dr. Burnham, whose remarks are also succinct and tremendously poignant.

A MINISTER LOOKS AT HEART PROBLEMS
The Reverend Dr. David H. Burnham

The pastor's experience describes far more than a résumé of education and church statistics. Particularly, it includes the adventure of living as well. Life is a walk. A classic writer described it as "Pilgrim's Progress."

My encounter with Nyles Reinfeld and the experiences I have shared with other heart patients don't provide simple slogans like "Chin up." Rather, they have taught me the importance of sensitivity, perspective, and patience. Lots of patience—because the heart patient feels and hears his heart. Heart difficulties may not be detected by the patient, but the rhythmic beat so long assumed—because of discovery or attack—now becomes a constant reminder of the beat of life.

The Lord Jesus has much to say about heart trouble: "Let not your heart be troubled . . . Neither let it be afraid." Of course, Christ was not simply referring to a physical organ or muscle function; He was describing the heart as the seat of personality—even as every student of Hebrew literature understood when David had written in Psalm 27. He spoke of God's strength so that "my heart shall not fear." These are two portions of scripture I regularly use with heart patients. I have learned the value of reading scripture, praying, and caring. My father had two open heart surgeries. He died following the second surgery without regaining consciousness. I have experienced the value of scripture, prayer, and care.

Since I was a junior in high school I have been aware of my own aortic insufficiency. I know firsthand about the heart, its effect on the spirit. I have learned patience, first with God and then with man. God has not designed me for heart failure, but something has caused disease and death. The Bible teaches that sin is the cause of death and that each of us has sinned. The Good News of Jesus Christ is that God can forgive us of our sins. By trusting in Jesus Christ and what He has done for us by dying on the cross for our sins, we can be forgiven and receive the gift of eternal life. Eternal life is not just "pie in the sky." It is having God's life and fellowship right now. Nothing is able to destroy or take that life away. Thus, to know that God cares so much that He sent His Son to die for me gives patience to my heart and spirit.

I have also learned patience with man. I don't fully understand why some persons have heart difficulties and others are spared, but I do know that when trouble comes we all react from our own point of reference. Having visited hospitals for over twenty-six years, I have seen evasion, joking, the appearance of indifference, anger, fear, confidence, and peace. In my visits I expect the spectrum, but I pray for the last two. That's why I visited Nyles—not at his request, as you have seen. Because it was unannounced, my visit lacked the opportunity to be more than just a last-chance cleric. Hence, even though I seek the opportunity for any meaningful chance to express compassion and concern, it rarely comes without personal invitation. The effect is too much like a stone hitting the windshield while driving at fifty-five miles an hour. Our tendency is to duck. So, unexpected visits can also cause people to duck. Nyles ducked and asked me to leave. I left his room sorry that we couldn't find at that time a place to meet heart and mind and just talk. I'm grateful that the chance has occurred at a later date. It is not often that someone doesn't want to pray, for the attitude of prayer usually represents at least concern. Nyles did not want an outsider's participation at that time, especially that of a preacher. However, he has since come to a conclusion that has left room for prayer and God's love. I believe this change has come through the character and love of his wife and children, who do care and pray. Nyles is on that pilgrim's walk to discover all that God has for his life in committing his life to Christ. I want to encourage his continued walk.

Pastoral visits are valuable because God cares, and so should we. Heart patients who have unexpected swings of temperament and spirit can be strengthened by our sensitivity and patience. I know. I hear my own heart beating.

Dr. Burnham has an almost endless amount of energy and compassion, as indicated by the freedom with which he gives his time to others. He was named pastor of the year in 1982 by the Moody Bible Institute.

9

"WAKE UP! THE OPERATION'S OVER!"

The induction room is the prep area for the operation. Here they install a number of leads into your body to provide information to the doctors and staff on the progress of your body functions.

Because you are put to sleep shortly after you enter the operating room and do not wake up again until several hours after the operation, you are completely unaware of what goes on during this stage. My information, therefore, on this intervening stage is provided by the clinic staff. For this purpose, the clinic assigned Mrs. Danni Nadler, R.N., to help me. Mrs. Nadler is another one of those petite, pretty nurses that seem to abound in hospitals. Why hospitals are so fortunate in this respect is only a matter of conjecture. It could be that medical functions attract large numbers of applicants and that doctors have a very discerning eye in their selections. I happen to think that what happens is that the qualities of tenderness and human compassion attract a certain type of beauty—beauty that could be as successful on the stage as in the mercy profession. These women certainly don't do it for the money. Although the nursing profession earns good money, it is not a high-income profession by any standards.

Mrs. Nadler's position was special consultant to patients and their families in the cardiovascular section. (Her own story appears in chapter 10.) She spent several days with me answering questions, and her help here and in many other portions of the book was invaluable. Parts of the book could not have been done without her assistance and, of course, the willing cooperation of the clinic. Throughout it all, the clinic and the staff in Akron were very helpful. There were no exceptions anywhere.

In the induction room you are greeted by a host of technical personnel. Each one begins attacking a certain part of your body: A catheter may be installed in your neck to measure pressures in your heart. This is also used for injecting medication. Another catheter is inserted in the wrist area, to act as an arterial mean to measure blood pressure. Monitor leads are attached to your arms near the chest to provide continuous ECGs.

While they are installing the neck catheter, a cloth is placed over your face. They didn't say why; they merely said it would be for a few minutes. To me this was the most frightening moment of the whole thing. I wanted to rip it off so I could see and breathe fresh air. I felt like I was in a coffin with the lid closed. My hands and legs were being strapped down, and now my face was covered up. (I learned later that the cloth covering was needed for purposes of sterility.) After a few moments, a nurse peaked in for a second, raising the cloth. "Is everything all right in there?" she asked to encourage me. Other patients must have felt my sense of panic at this moment.

I remember no more. I was asleep. The sodium pentothol had entered one of the catheters and was circulating in my blood.

In the meantime, my family had departed to the family lounge. Here a hostess talks with the family and tells them to have breakfast or lunch. They are given a packet of papers to read. Following surgery, the doctor sees them and then has them go home or to the hotel. They are called if a problem develops. Heart operations of this type usually last from three to six hours, but the actual duration is difficult to predict, depending upon the complexity and any difficulties that are encountered.

From the induction room, you are moved into the operating room.

Here they install a breathing tube, which is inserted in the mouth and passes down the throat between the vocal cords into the lungs. A catheter is installed into the bladder to keep it drained and to monitor kidney functions. The skin is prepped with an antiseptic soap solution and the body covered with sterile drapes.

A team of surgeons and surgical technicians makes the chest incision and removes the vein from the leg. This vein is the same one removed from people with varicose veins.

Since my left leg had already been stripped for my previous operation, they now used the vein from the right leg. To
remove it, the doctors made interrupted incisions from the
ankle to the groin. They also used a mammary artery from the
left side of the chest wall. (Since they've swiped so many of
my spare parts, I don't know where they'll get replacements
the next time, if they need them.) The mammary artery is
smaller than the leg vein; although it passes less blood, it is
pulsatile and has the advantage over the leg vein in that it
plugs up less readily. As I mentioned earlier, my leg-vein
bypass had sealed itself off completely. That's why I was back
for seconds. This time the doctors felt that the mammary
artery would give more permanent relief. Whereas the first
operation was good for six years, this one should be good for
ten or more.

The chest incision runs down the center of the chest and
is about ten inches long. (At one time, when this type of
operation healed up, you looked like you had a zipper in your
chest from the stitches, and people with heart operations used
to refer to themselves as members of the "zipper club." The
Cleveland Clinic Foundation, and many others, now use sub-
cutaneous stitches that eliminate this effect.) After the incision, the rib bones are opened up like a bomb-bay door. The
mammary artery is then dissected from the chest wall, and
one end is cut and inserted into the heart area. Repeat operations take longer because of old scar tissue and also because of
the wires that were used to hold your ribs together the first
time. Old heart pacer wires also may be left over from the past.
These are now removed.

You are next hooked up to the heart machine. Your own
heart is stopped. This means that by pre-1960 standards you
are now dead. The heart machine, hooked into your atrium
and aorta, takes over the pumping action for your heart. This
phase lasts about an hour or so, since most of the operating
time is spent in opening and closing.

While on the machine, the body is cooled down to protect the heart muscle. A chemical solution is administered to
reduce metabolism and protect the body.

Coming off the heart machine is the most critical time of

the operation. This is when the work is turned back to the patient. The heart may not always want to take back all of the work—depending on past stresses and damage.

When the bypasses, or other operations on the heart, are completed, the surgical team dries up the operation site and makes sure that nothing is oozing or bleeding. Most heart bypass operations are surprisingly efficient, with little loss of blood. The patient may not require a transfusion of blood at all, as his own blood is given back to him by means of a blood-salvage system. Clotting chemicals are given to counteract previous chemicals given to prevent clotting. Pacemaking wires are commonly installed. These come in sets of two to four wires. The wires are inserted under the surface of the heart muscle (the heart has no skin). Chest tubes are installed to drain blood out of the chest cavity. These usually involve two to four plastic tubes that stick out of your chest. None of these tubes runs into the stomach. They look like they do, and I suppose I thought that they did because I expected to be deathly sick to my stomach when I awoke; when I wasn't, I thought one of these tubes was draining my stomach. Instead, the stomach is drained through a nasal-gastric tube that passes through the nose and into the stomach. This tube is installed at the same time as the breathing tube.

The chest is closed by wiring the sternum together and closing the skin, using special stitches. These stitches dissolve in a few days and do not need to be removed. In fact, the only stitches that had to be removed, in my case, were those holding the pacemaker wires. The pacemaker wires are a precaution that is used as a standby should a pacemaker be needed to stabilize the heart rhythm.

The leg incision is closed at the same time as the chest.

You are now transferred to a bed and wheeled to the intensive care unit.

In the intensive care (or recovery) unit, the various body functions are monitored and stabilized. Medications are adjusted according to the readings. You are still on the breathing machine, which took over your breathing at the start of the anesthesia. Your body is still paralyzed and asleep.

As the medication wears off, usually in a few hours, the body begins to do its own work.

Several times during the awakening period, a nurse leans over, addresses you by name, and says, "The surgery is over." This is meant to reassure you and orient you to your status. My reaction reminded me of my earlier comment about being awakened to get a sleeping pill. Why wake me up to tell me that? I thought to myself. I just wanted to sleep. In all likelihood, the nurse hadn't wakened me at all, but rather had seen me stirring. I really was glad to know.

Another disturbing experience occurs at this time. As you begin to wake up and take over your own duties, you suddenly can't breathe. I got the nurse's attention somehow, and she leaned over. In the preoperative training class they had told us to talk to the nurse by printing on the palm of her hand with a finger—only the key word, spelled with capital letters. With the tubes in your mouth and nose, talking was impossible. To get the message across I tried writing on my palm but that didn't work. She held out her own hand and I tried writing I CANT BREATHE!

But it was too long for her. So I erased it with a flip of my hand and wrote BREATH. "You can't breathe?" she asked. I nodded, jubilant at the success of our partnership. I had learned a new way to communicate. I had done this once on a trip to Mexico, communicating out of a dictionary. I now had established communication with the world.

"You can't breathe because you're fighting the machine," she said in a mean voice, or at least it seemed unsympathetic to me. I fell asleep instantly, worn out by my long stay in the world of the living, wondering how not to fight the machine.

I awoke again, out of breath. The same thing happened, but I was smarter this time. I wasted no time, but went straight to the word BREATH.

"You can't breathe?" she asked again. I nodded again, noting my improvement in communications, if not in breathing. "You're fighting the machine," she said again, like we were playing a broken record. I waited for her to explain, half asleep, half afraid to go to sleep.

"You've got to breathe *with* the machine, not against it. When it's exhaling," she went on, explaining the process, "you're inhaling. Do like it does. Breathe with it." How, I wondered do I find out about this marvelous machine? How do I learn when it wants to inhale? I fell asleep again, confused and tormented by my doubts. What if I couldn't learn this trick? It scared me with its implications. Why didn't they give me a smarter machine? One that did what I did?

A little later—seconds later, perhaps—a man's voice cut through the hazy world of my sleep-saturated mind. "When you hear the buzzer, take a deep breath," the voice said. He sounded so confident that I believed him and felt my problem was solved. I knew now what to do. They had learned of my problem and rigged up a buzzer for me, I thought, my heart soaring.

I listened carefully and heard a buzzer. I took a deep breath. Then another buzzer went off. Then still another. The room was full of buzzers! Everyone in the room was on a breathing machine. Which one was mine? I listened attentively. One of the buzzers seemed slightly louder. That must be mine, my analytical mind informed me. So I latched onto it and breathed faithfully in rhythm to its friendly buzzer. The voice spoke up reassuringly. "You're doing fine," it said. I wasn't so sure. Every once in a while I would fall alseep and lose my buzzer. I wanted him to stay close by till I got the hang of it.

I was still unsure of myself when they dealt me a new blow. "We're going to take you off the respirator," a friendly lady nurse informed me. I wanted to get off and make progress, I thought to myself. But what if I haven't learned yet how to breathe? What happens if I fall asleep? They kept telling me to stay awake during it all, and I kept falling asleep. "Stay awake!" they'd order me sharply. Then I'd fall asleep again. "You were asleep again," the voice would cut in, scolding me. I felt so guilty about it all, but I couldn't stay awake. Then I fell asleep and got a good rest. No one bothered me.

Somewhere in this stretch of time my wife and daughter came to see me. I remember the visit only vaguely, if at all. Since close relatives are allowed in the intensive care unit about thirty-six hours after the operation, the sequence of my memory is twisted out of shape. This disorientation is not unexpected. It is difficult to keep track of time in an area where the lights are on twenty-four hours a day and where there is continuous activity. In that setting, the senses can be misleading. You become confused. This confusion tends to be worse at night than during the day.

Medication given for pain also increases the likelihood of disorientation. This temporary confusion, if it occurs, is not serious and quickly resolves itself within a day or two after you are transferred to a more restful unit. As rest is achieved, normal patterns of sleep, wakefulness, and thought return.

More vivid in my memory than my family's visit was the patient on the bed beside me. He woke up screaming and shouting. He woke me too. He jumped up on his bed and pulled the hoses out of his chest. They were trying to kill him, he shouted. They told him his wife and family were at his side, but he wouldn't believe anyone. This happened several times. Then a nurse came over to my bed and said they had moved him across the room so I could get some rest. At times I woke up and could see him across the room, still trying to get free from the staff. The experience was disturbing, not only because of my own weakness, but also because I wondered if I might go out of my mind like that.

These experiences are not rare with any type of serious surgery. They occur because the patient is reduced to almost total dependence. For people who are accustomed to dominating others, it is an experience with which they have trouble coping. As the anesthesia wears off, there is a short time in which patients may not have regained the ability to move their arms or legs. There is a time before the mind and body become coordinated. Although to me this poor man's terror seemed to be a disaster for him, Mrs. Nadler says such patients recover their mental balance as they progress and recover from the operation without ill effects. The human body survives against unbelievable odds in its fight to live.

As I recall the incident, I wonder how much of it was real and how much of it I might have dreamed. Since the body is completely discoordinated, and talking is impossible without removing the tube in the throat, it is very unlikely that the patient could have done all of these things.

The situation reminds me of a case involving a friend who suffered a severe heart attack. His heart stopped, and the emergency staff hit him several times with a defibrillator and took other emergency measures. The doctors finally announced that it was no use. The man was dead.

My friend, on the other hand, was totally aware of the activity in the room. He felt like he was outside of his own body and could look down at the scene, seeing even himself. He kept shouting, "It's not too late! I'm still alive! Try again!"

Fortunately for him, they did try again, and his heart began to beat. He now moves about as freely as you and I and would scarcely seem to be a man who was once thought dead. This was two years ago.

Could some of those cries of anguish that I heard have been coming from deep inside of my own body as I lay immobile, while my conscious mind began to stir?

I recall no similar experiences with my first operation, so I can't really answer. The incident seemed to be extended over a period of hours, and it recurred with a patient on the seventh floor after I had been moved there. Hence, reality and imagination may easily have been interchanged in those dim hours.

Two more cases of this type have since come to my attention. This time I was able to get the picture with a clear mind, on a return visit to the clinic three months later.

The first case involved a man of approximately fifty-five who was a "re-op" (in clinic terminology; "back for seconds" in my own untutored patois). His first operation was in 1978, some four years earlier. For several days after he returned to the postoperative care unit, he continued to hallucinate. He thought he was back having his old operation. He thought it was 1978. He even thought he was in a hospital in his home town. The clinic sent several specialists to help him regain his orientation, including Mrs. Nadler.

His problem was resolved before he left the clinic, but the next case has some sad overtones.

The second man was sixty-six and a devout Catholic, with a strong military background as well. He thought he was being held captive in a concentration camp. (In his own life, he had never been a prisoner of war, but somehow he associated his clinic experiences with what he assumed to be the conditions of a concentration camp.) For his own protection, he had to be restrained; his arms were tied down.

Many patients who hallucinate visualize themselves being assaulted sexually or being tortured, or they exhibit some other distortion of basic human drives. Religion often creates hidden conflicts that erupt to the surface in times like these, as do other aggressive tendencies, such as I mentioned earlier.

This man's problems were exacerbated by his critical condition at the time he arrived at the clinic. When he was admitted he was suffering from a very serious heart problem. His heart had developed a hole, and he wasn't expected to live. He, himself, was reconciled to dying when they brought him in. The failing condition of the heart in turn caused his liver to malfunction, and the consequent poisoning of his system very likely intensified or triggered many of his hallucinations.

Although the man's physical recovery was clearly a miracle of modern surgery, his hallucinations lingered up to the time he was discharged. But even here, considerable progress had been made.

First-time bypass patients are usually moved to the seventh floor after the breathing tube is removed. Repeat patients, like myself, are held longer for observation, usually an extra night.

When the breathing tube is removed, you are given an oxygen face tube to wear. This hangs over your ears like a pair of glasses, with a short tube in each nostril. This stays on for one day after you go to the seventh floor.

While you are still in intensive care, you are given personal responsibility for asking for pain relief. You can now receive ice chips to suck on. The bladder tube comes out. This is a funny sensation. There is no pain involved, but you feel like your lower insides have been exhausted through a vacuum cleaner. The tight wrappings that have bound your legs are removed. The dressings on the chest incision are removed and replaced with small patches. The pressure lines are removed from your wrist. The gastric tube has been removed with the breathing tube, and the chest tubes are extracted.

Again the sensation is more like your inner chest has been vacuumed than one of pain. There is very little pain involved in removing any of these tubes or attachments.

Once you are breathing on your own, they make you sit up, and the breathing exercise begins. Sitting up and holding a pillow to your chest, they pound or tap your back and tell you to cough. "Cough harder!" they tell you. You do your best, so they'll let you lie down again and go to sleep.

Sleep is the most precious commodity you have in that ward, and they keep taking it from you. You breathe into the breathing tube, inhale as hard as you can to pull the ball to the top of the tube. You hold it as long as you can. Your lungs want to break. You repeat this several times. Then they pound you again and you cough. Finally, the therapist says, "Very good. You're doing real well." And you lay down and go back to sleep. This goes on every two hours or so.

These deep-breathing exercises and coughing are, as we saw earlier, important steps to recovery. Coughing not only reduces the chances of pneumonia, but it also reduces the incidence of fever. It does not actually disturb the incision in the chest or the bypass grafts. It is also nowhere near as violent as I have suggested; it only seems that way to the patient. Actually, the therapist clasps both hands against the side of your chest, and this action causes vibrations within the lungs that loosen the secretions, making them easier to cough up.

Changing your position on the bed, from side to side and onto the back, is also an aid in this respect. Lying too long on your back allows the secretions to collect in the lungs.

With these accomplishments under your belt, you are now ready for the seventh floor.

"Can I have 7Q?" I asked the male nurse. "I think you can," he answered. At last I was on my way out of the world of sleep and fog and into a bright new world.

They helped me step from the bed to the floor and into a wheelchair. Then, sitting up with an IV still sticking in my neck and the oxygen tubes in my nose, I was wheeled through the halls and elevated to the seventh floor. As unit ward 7Q loomed into sight, my heart and imagination jumped for joy.

10
CARDIOVASCULAR COUNSELING

THE HUMAN SIDE OF THE HOSPITAL
Danni Gogol Nadler, R.N.

(Note: Prior to becoming the Cardiovascular Counselor at the Cleveland Clinic Foundation, Mrs. Nadler, the nurse mentioned in the previous chapter, served in various cardiovascular units at the clinic as a practicing nurse.)

Cardiovascular counseling at the clinic evolved to meet the needs of the patient and the family.

It grew out of a recognition that both the patient and the family often feel a sense of isolation as they are absorbed into the hospital routine. This feeling may result in part from the fragmentation and inconsistency of trust relationships that evolve around the patient. For example, doctors are not always available to spend as much time as is necessary for "rehashing" experiences, feelings, thoughts, fears, and concerns. Although the physician has the ultimate control and responsibility for the patient's well-being; it may be difficult for the patient and family to "risk all" in talking to the doctor. The aura of "the doctor" may make it difficult for them even to listen and hear what he has to say. Because they want the doctors and nurses to like them, they may fear that what they say will be viewed as a challenge.

Furthermore, there is often much more going on within a family unit than initially presents itself. These factors affect not only what is perceived but also what information is needed about the patient's situation. The counselor's presence is therefore important in order to increase their sense of security and to reduce feelings of panic and frustration. The counselor becomes a trusted friend who can answer questions and provide a helping hand for coming to grips with the situation. When this type of understanding is missing, the result can produce serious reactions that can be triggered by a

125

relatively minor event. If this happens, the stage is set for a bad hospital experience regardless of the outcome.

When patients or their families are threatened and fearful, anything that is said or done may heighten these fears. Any apparent insensitivity may be perceived as a threat. Because patients and families come to the hospital with varying degrees of knowledge, understanding, and acceptance of their disease, interpretation of the patient's condition may differ from one member to another. It is important, therefore, to determine as quickly as possible the extent of their understanding, so that an ongoing process of improving their knowledge can be instituted. Cardiovascular counseling is not only concerned with the immediate crisis situation but must also help the patient resolve the long-term implications of a chronic disease.

The purpose, therefore, of counseling is to help each family member perceive the illness in such a way that they will be emotionally ready to move on to a better understanding and acceptance of the future, so that they can enjoy optimal health and well-being.

A counseling relationship can be initiated at any point during the course of a patient's illness. Perhaps the ideal time is when the need for catheterization has been determined.

Basically, all patients need some degree of emotional preparation. Counseling can help reduce patients' anxiety about the cardiac catheterization and at the same time prepare them for the possibility of surgery. Naturally, the amount of counseling needed depends upon the patient's condition at the time he or she enters the hospital. Patients with a long history of heart problems obviously need less immediate help than those who have been struck down suddenly. To patients who have been walking around feeling good just a few days before, who have been completely active with no limitations, the sudden prospect of having an invasive test performed or of having their hearts operated on is awesome. These patients find it difficult to listen to what is being explained to them. They are the ones who often need a counselor to repeat what has been discussed by the physician and to explore their feelings and questions about the procedures that lie ahead of them. Patients experiencing unrelenting chest pain or in the throes of a catastrophe feel very close to death and find it difficult to listen to much of anything. They just want help. Recall of what has been said to these patients is often vague. Postcatheterization and postsurgery explanations are thus more meaningful to them than what they hear before. Patients who face surgery for disease in the vessels of the leg or the neck, for example, often find it difficult to understand why they need tests on the heart and may possibly need heart surgery as well. Both patients with such seemingly unrelated problems and patients in for a routine checkup need a lot of emotional preparation. It is a very difficult time for their families also, since nothing may be making a whole lot of sense to them. It is difficult for them to shift their focus from one health problem to another. Patients who face a reoperation usually start out feeling disappointed—if not depressed— about the fact that they are now "in trouble again." Prior to the recatheterization they may delude themselves into thinking that everything is fine, as long as they are not having chest pain. Once they are catheterized, however, reality becomes fact. This can be a very difficult time for them, particularly if the first experience was not a good one.

It is therefore very helpful for a counselor to be available to these people—whether surgery is indicated electively, urgently, or on an emergency basis. The counselor begins by letting the family and patient know that he or she will keep in regular contact with them. Events and decisions often move rapidly; once patients are in the hospital, they may express feelings of walking in the dark. Informative programs, which may be available at the hospital, are often overlooked or ignored. They need someone to guide them or tell them which program to watch. Patients and families usually set the pace for the counselor. They let the counselor know their need for information, the fears that they have and want to discuss, their need for denial, and their concerns for the future. Having a counselor present when the cardiologist discusses the cath and makes recommendations to the patient and the family establishes the counselor as a backup resource who has heard exactly what they have heard and can confirm or reinterpret the information for them.

One of the most difficult times for patients and families

alike is the interim between catheterization and the operation. Once the need for surgery has been confirmed, it lies like a lead weight on all of them. They find it difficult to concentrate on anything else. This is the time when patient and family may express thoughts about what they might have done to alter the course of events. At this time, they need someone to help them put back into perspective the fact that history cannot be changed and that they must instead begin to deal with the future. The first step along this route is the surgery itself. When surgery is just a day or two away, patients and their families usually are unable to listen or learn much about the disease or its future management. The anxiety and excitement surrounding the surgery are too great. For patients who may need to wait several weeks or months before the operation, this interim provides an excellent time to discuss the disease process, its natural history, and risk-factor control. Part of the question about what could have been done to alter the state of affairs is "why me?" Though no one has the complete answer to the cause of coronary artery disease, part of the answer is in risk factors. Learning about the disease process, how it occurs, and the role the risk factors play gives the patient a sense of control over the management of the disease. Furthermore, heart disease is a family problem. The earlier the patient and family recognize, understand, and accept this fact, the more capable they will be in dealing with it. People in their thirties and forties and very assertive, controlling individuals find it especially difficult to face up to their situation. It is hard for them to accept a disease that can significantly shorten their life span. Yet they often accept the surgery itself with little trouble. They react almost as if they were bargaining or trading their future: "You take the disease away and I'll take the surgery." It is important at this time to avoid allowing patients to delude themselves into believing that after surgery, they will be "fixed," will be "as good as new," will "have a new heart," or will never have any more trouble. The truth should be maintained and reinforced in spite of the patients' or families' inability to listen or accept the fact that they are dealing with a permanent and progressive disease. At some point they start asking questions about the disease and the function of their heart in relation to their life style and future life span. These questions often occur after surgery, before discharge from the hospital. Usually it is the counselor, who responds to their concerns. Once patients have had surgery they can no longer deny that something is wrong—seriously wrong—otherwise there would be no need for anything as major and dramatic as open heart surgery. Following surgery, they are weakened and somewhat demoralized, and they are ready to listen, even if they don't like what they hear. Usually, if time permits, a relationship has been established with the patient by the doctors and other professionals prior to the operation, so that anything that needs to be said will have been said before. This can help patients and families accept the state of affairs. They can be made to understand that their situation is not hopeless, that there are choices to be made and things that can be done to help, that they have some control over their future. The future can be as happy as they make it. Furthermore, there are other important prospects for the future. For example, there may be exciting new ways of treating and managing cardiovascular disease on the horizon. After all, only fifteen years ago we could not do anything at all to alter the mechanical obstruction.

Special counseling is required for those patients who have very little or no chest pain and have suffered no restrictions on their activity. It is extremely important that these patients understand what is going on and why surgery is indicated. Surgery will not make them feel better, since they were not disabled or uncomfortable to begin with. All they will see and feel is the bill. Since open heart surgery is not cheap, the fact of not feeling better could lead to misunderstanding and resentment. In a case such as this, the patient needs to understand that the issues are basic ones of life and death. The decisions involved are based on statistics of groups of individuals who have had similar arterial blockages and suffered serious consequences that could have been treated. What bypass surgery offers these patients is protection against a possible catastrophic event (major heart attack or death) in the near future.

Though the risk of routine open heart surgery is very low (around 1 percent), it is not zero. An individual's risk will vary with the specifics of the disease, heart function, and other medical problems. Risk of operation should be specifically and directly discussed with each patient and family. Risks are also relative to the alternative: what is likely to happen without surgery. For some patients, the risk of not having surgery may be certain death or disability. In those cases the risks imposed by the surgical procedure will always be lower, regardless of how high they are intrinsically, and surgery represents the only logical choice. These points need to be established and understood. Furthermore, risk of surgery is not limited to death alone, even though death may be the patient's main concern. What may not be considered are the risks of complications, the most difficult of which is the stroke. This risk should be discussed with every patient, even if there is no particular reason to think that he or she is under any greater risk than anyone else. This is the one complication that has not been controlled or reduced very much, despite all the advances and the reduction in the overall risk.

Reoperations involve a higher risk than primary operations (around 3 to 5 percent). There are a number of reasons for this. First, reoperations are more difficult to perform because of adhesions (scar tissue)—all the tissues in the chest are stuck together. Second, it takes longer to do these operations. This means usually a longer anesthetic time and pump run (time on the heart-lung machine). Third, the patient is usually several years older, and something has taken place to put the patient in jeopardy again. The hospital course may not be the same as the first time. Patients may need to be in the intensive care unit longer and may not get back on their feet as fast. Usually, the first and second operation involve different hospital experiences, even if the same hospital and same surgeon are used and the two operations occur relatively close together. This doesn't mean one is better or worse necessarily, just different. The patient's memory of the events can be different, even though the sequence and the actual events may have been the same. Both patients and families seem to weather their experiences better if all these elements have been discussed with them.

At the Cleveland Clinic Foundation, patients often don't meet the surgeon until the evening before surgery. It is usually at this time also that they meet the counselor, who sits in on the discussions between the doctor and the patient. This meeting establishes the counselor's credibility with the family and patient and is critical to the relationship that follows. The family learns that it can turn to the counselor for help or advice at any time of the day or night.

Patient and family attend a breathing and a pre-op class the evening before surgery. A respiratory therapist teaches the patient the importance of lung function and how to perform the breathing treatment after surgery. An intensive care nurse explains what both the patient and the family can expect for the next few days. Counseling takes place with the patient and family again after the classes and again after they have talked with the surgeon to clarify any last-minute questions. At the Cleveland Clinic, since about fifteen open heart surgeries are performed a day, not everyone can be operated on first thing in the morning. If the patient is not going first, I, as the counselor, will stop in in the morning before he or she must go down to surgery. Waiting on the day of surgery is probably one of the most difficult and anxious times for the patient. (Waiting to know how the patient is doing during the operation is one of the most difficult and anxious times for the family.) Once the patient is medicated, the day of surgery is the patient's easy day—there is nothing to do but sleep the whole day. By contrast, for the family this is usually a very long and emotionally exhausting day. Once the patient is clinically stable, he or she needs to start working. The patient starts hurting and feels exhausted, while the family is able to relax and go back to some type of normal living.

What seems to be helpful and comforting to both patient and family is to have the counselor in the operating room during the patient's surgery—someone who will periodically talk with the family so that they know at all times how the patient is doing. Because my relationship has been established, they trust me to tell them exactly what is happening, making it easier for them to cope with the waiting. It also enables them to listen and understand more fully what the surgeon will be telling them once the operation has been completed. Again, I am present when the surgeon speaks with them about the surgical outcome, the patient's condition, the anticipated hospital course, and so on. It is important for me to hear what is said on both sides so that in the future I can validate what was actually said. It must be remembered that the patient is not present and may need some objective confirmation that what the family tells him is actually what was said.

Keeping the family up-to-date on the events in surgery is especially valuable if there are complications. It helps prepare them for any eventuality. All the time and effort spent in developing a relationship and educating the patient and family prior to surgery pays enormous dividends should a complicated hospital course become a reality. The trust relationship is of immeasurable value during a time of crisis. People usually understand the possibility that complications or death may occur in the operating room. Though families are anxious during the patient's operation, they are probably better prepared to listen and accept the possibility of complications and even death at that time than at any other time during the hospitalization. Please do not misunderstand: I do not mean that the loss is any less, nor do I mean that it is easy to accept; I mean that their ability to cope and deal realistically with the situation is better.

Intraoperative difficulties fall into several categories:

1. Technical (in which it is anatomically difficult to do the surgery because of the patient's structures, adhesions, tissue integrity, lack of adequate vein, etc.)
2. Bleeding problems
3. Inadequate or insufficient heart function
4. End-organ dysfunction (kidneys and lungs in particular)

Difficulties such as these can be discussed with the family during the operation, as well as how the problems are being managed. Acceptance of the outcome is enhanced if the family understands that there may not be a simple solution. If the problems are resolved, the situation is easily accepted, and the time spent in explaining does not seem to have been in vain. The family's overall understanding of the situation is broadened. If problems persist into the postoperative period, or if the patient does not survive, the family can face that outcome with some basic understanding of the events leading to it. Being kept abreast of all the events that are taking place helps the family's ability to listen to the surgeon when explaining and summarizing the operative course. My presence serves not only to support and reassure the family but also to help them begin dealing with their grief. One of the greatest services I can offer a family is to assist them in mobilizing their resources, to continue life's functioning in the midst of tremendous loss. Because of the long-standing trust relationship, I can be a friend and a professional who is able to offer guidance and share in reexploring feelings in relation to our previous discussions.

The evening of surgery often brings a very long night for the family, particularly if the patient underwent surgery early that day. In the evening report, I can either verify that the patient is stable or can initiate information about complications that may be evolving. Because of the risk of stroke, I always let the family know if the patient has awakened from the anesthesia. I also review what they need to do next to get information about the patient and when they can expect to hear from me again.

I'd like to return to my earlier statement about being personally available to the patient or family at any time, to whatever degree they deem necessary. This type of commitment is most often tested when there are complications or if death seems imminent, as in the event of emergency surgery, problems during surgery, reopens (going back to the operating room because of bleeding or poor heart function), and cardiac or respiratory arrest (either in the intensive care unit or on the regular nursing floor). These, obviously, are physical problems. There are also mental and emotional problems that require special attention. The two most common of these are situations that revolve around "post-op psychosis" (basically confusion, paranoia, and belligerence) and tragic events that occur around the time of the patient's operation (such as the death, serious illness, or injury of another family member).

Problems have an uncanny way of occurring at odd hours of the night or morning. Weekends and holidays also seem to be a favorite time for mishaps. Actually, that probably isn't so;

it just seems that way. When unexpected situations arise during the day, when everyone is awake and at hand ready to help, people feel more secure. That's the time when things are supposed to be taken care of, the time for work to be done. Night time is for rest. At night, people are less oriented and rational. They need that time to regenerate their own resources. Weekends and holidays are for other things—enjoyment, relaxation, pleasant things.

If what I do is of any value, it comes to fruition during those out-of-ordinary times. A case in point: The patient has been doing fine during his operation, so the family has gone home for a few hours. Then the patient begins to bleed. In my evening call, I let the family know he's bleeding and the possibility of his needing to go back to the operating room. They automatically feel the need to rush back to the hospital. This would mean not being able to reach them because they would be in transit. Furthermore, there's a chance that they might get into trouble themselves (they most likely would not be concentrating on their driving). Their panic often has to do with being afraid they will not know what is happening. They need to be reassured of periodic contact. It's best for them to stay safe at home, where they can be kept up-to-date. They can accept this advice more easily if they know I will stay at the hospital to keep the vigil for them; knowing I will not leave allows them to stay home and listen. How long it takes for situations to settle down varies from a few hours into the evening to the wee hours of the morning. In another example, a patient was admitted as an emergency myocardial infarction (MI), and turned out to have a dissecting aorta. He was deteriorating rapidly. He needed something now. But what to do and how to do it wasn't perfectly clear, nor was his chance of survival. His situation was such that he was going to die unless we were able to help him. His operation began at 7 P.M. Friday, after an already full operating day, and didn't end until 7 A.M. Saturday. During those twelve hours, as problems developed and were resolved, the family and I discussed all the events of the past, present, and possible future. Though the patient's hospital course was long and rocky, there was never any time when the patient or the family felt alone, neglected, or in the dark. The entire hospital course became a good learning experience.

Let me tell you about one of my most treasured experiences. A patient with valvular heart disease had a fairly routine valve replacement. After a few months he returned to have the valve re-replaced because of a developing infection on the valve. His surgery was done on a semiemergency basis. He subsequently went on to have a total of six open heart operations in a span of two years. Roughly every three months, on an emergency basis (in the middle of the night and on weekends), we replaced one or two valves—not because the valves malfunctioned but because the tissue in his heart didn't hold. These are problems we cannot fix. Such desire to live, such understanding of the inevitable, and such immense courage to accept and deal with the situation by both the patient and family truly made me a better person. Though I know they feel very close and grateful to me for always being there to guide and support them, I doubt it will ever compare to the lessons in life they gave to me—to all of us.

When patients are very ill, they know better than anyone else what their situation is. If they are able to respond and talk, they usually are very grateful to have someone to talk to, someone who understands their situation and recognizes how ill they are. If the family can be helped to let the patient know that they also understand the situation, what needs to be said on both sides can be said without false pretenses. If death ensues, the dying experience is more peaceful and better.

Death is the last inevitable experience we all have. The timing is almost never good—but none of us can choose the time. It is my experience that patients very often know they are going to die. Sometimes they know before surgery, and they actually try to prepare their family. Most often the family refuses to hear what is being said. As a result, it's often easier for the patient to tell me and have me tell the family. If they tell me before surgery, I find I can't talk them out of the operation. Even to their own doctors they will deny feeling that they are going to die. But they do know, and they are always right.

It is not that they want to die, nor that they decide they will die; it is more like a given knowledge. They are not afraid, although they may be angry because it is not of their own choosing and they don't want to leave their family. The stage at which people reach this knowledge varies. Sometimes they know before surgery, sometimes after, but they always know. This sense of finality is very different from being afraid to die or of facing death as a possibility. It is a given, accepted knowledge, and I always listen when they tell me. It is much easier for the family to deal with death when they know the patient is reconciled to it. None of us can escape death. But how it is experienced by the patient and family affects how well the family goes on living. I said it was a privilege to see a patient and family through a crisis, but the greatest privilege of all is to share in bridging the transition from life to death, to help the family go on living with a loss.

Probably one of the toughest parts for the family is seeing an extremely ill patient who seems to be having a lot of pain. Generally, patients who are extremely ill do not have a great deal of pain, though they may be uncomfortable. It seems that nature has a way of protecting us when there is too much to deal with by stopping us from interpreting it. Patients who have been extremely ill tell me not only that they don't remember having much pain but also that they have a very difficult time recalling anything at all. Time itself has very little relevance to anything. Time, sequence of events, and physical feeling only seem to take on significance when the patient is getting better. This is when everyone else begins to relax and feel better. Hence, it is easier for the family to deal with the knowledge that a patient is not feeling well if they know he or she is at least *doing* well. On the other hand, if the patient is not getting well, it helps to know that he or she is not suffering.

Emergencies also tend to be tougher on families than on patients. Most often emergencies for heart patients are thought of in terms of surgery. Emergency operations are done for a number of reasons. Sometimes, what starts out as a routine heart catheterization ends with the patient in the operating room because of irretractable chest pain, arrhythmia (irregular heartbeat—usually ventricular), or pump failure (inability of the heart to work effectively or efficiently enough to sustain life). Like any emergency, this has real shock value for both the patient and the family; they were prepared only for a test, not a major life-threatening operation. Even transluminal coronary angioplasty (dilating the area of obstruction in the coronary artery with a balloon at the end of the catheter during catheterization) sometimes fails, and the patient needs to go directly to surgery. The possibility of surgery is discussed with the patient and family prior to the procedure, so that the idea is not new and the sense of emergency and shock are reduced. Emergency operations may also arise when a patient has acute chest pain, perhaps for the first time, and goes to the hospital. The doctor may feel that the patient is in the throes of a heart attack. The doctor starts some intravenous medications and whisks him off to the cath lab for a catheterization. From there, the patient may go directly to the operating room, if one or more critical lesions (blockages) have been found. This situation obviously does not allow time for "getting used to the idea." None of the events was even entertained, let alone planned for. The thought of having a disease may be totally foreign to both patient and family. Sometimes emergencies arise while the patient is in the hospital. If there is an increase in the amount or severity of chest pain or the ECG changes, it may warrant surgery earlier than planned. Postoperative emergencies can also arise. Occasionally patients need to go back to the operating room the night of surgery or the next day because of bleeding—which is usually not difficult to correct. Sometimes the patient may go into cardiac arrest and need to have the chest reopened regardless of where he or she is—in the intensive care unit, on the regular nursing floor, or in the room. Obviously, the patient must go back to the operating room at least to have the chest closed.

Emergencies do not always require surgery. On occasion, patients have problems—such as respiratory difficulties, arrhythmias, end-organ dysfunctions (most often the kidneys), or neurologic deficits (most commonly stroke)—on the regular nursing floor and need to go back to the intensive care unit.

Regardless of the reason for the emergency, certain reactions are universal. There is a sense of shock and disbelief. I find the family needs to be sat down and "talked to." They listen best if I am physically at their level and use continual eye contact. I talk slowly and repeat the facts a number of times. Almost always panic sets in to some degree. The response to the panic is (1) to find something to do to change the situation, (2) to gather reinforcements, or (3) to run away from the problems. Usually none of these responses is carefully thought out or valuable. Families become extremely dependent and vulnerable. Though people generally can make decisions that are best for them, they need a great deal of honest and factual information and objective guidance so that all aspects of the situation are kept in perspective. There is a tendency for families to respond in one of two fashions: broadcasting or blackout. Either they call everyone and have all these other people come and take care of everything that has happened or ever will happen, or else they don't let anyone—not even the patient—know anything and put everything on hold so that nothing bad can ever happen again. (Of course I am oversimplifying and exaggerating a little.)

There are also external crises that affect the patient, things that may have nothing at all to do with the patient's physical state. There is a tendency for people to feel that other terrible things cannot happen if they are already dealing with a major event like open heart surgery. People are so consumed that they stop seeing the rest of the world. Unfortunately, the rest of the world may include such things as problems with the business, the home burning down, an injury to a child, or the death of a spouse. Families are to some degree on guard and brace themselves to hear bad news about the patient, but they are totally unprepared to hear about other bad news. It's like hitting them with a lead balloon. Typically they respond irrationally. It's the "straw that broke the camel's back." If they have been coping up to that point, that usually ends it. Here's an example:

An out-of-state patient came with his wife for bypass surgery. They happened to have very close friends and relatives in town for the wife to stay with. The patient's children also came from out of town. The day before surgery I received a frantic call from the patient's son saying his mother had suffered a heart attack and was in another Cleveland hospital. He wanted all calls to his father's room stopped. He wanted his father to know nothing of the event until after his operation. I asked the son if he didn't think his father would wonder why his wife wasn't visiting and why no one was calling. He said he would tell him she had a cold and that they didn't want people bothering him. The son and family had discussed everything (or so they thought) and felt adamant about wanting to protect the patient from being upset and worried about his wife because it might interfere with how well he would survive the operation.

Obviously, the family's motives were good. They loved the patient and didn't want him hurt. What they didn't think about was the patient's right to know. Nor did they think about the possible sequence of future events. When situations like this occur, people do not want it to be true. So they go to great length trying to keep it from being a reality to everyone. They try to solve the immediate event and close their eyes to the possibility of any ramifications or consequences.

After a very long, arduous discussion exploring the possible long-term effect of how the situation was handled, the family conceded to trust my judgment in telling the patient about his wife's heart attack, not only prior to his surgery but right away. The overwhelming reason for telling the patient was that he had the right to know and to make the decision that he could ultimately live best with knowing all the facts and possibilities. The biggest factor to consider is that the possible outcome for one or the other is death (for the patient during surgery, for the wife, from an extension of her MI). But the patient and his wife may have important things to say to each other. To take that chance away from them by making the decision not to tell the husband the facts is a right the family does not have. Most of the time things get better: The patient has his surgery, and the wife recovers from her heart attack without incident. That is what the family assumed would happen. But that is not an appropriate line of reasoning.

Patients generally respond more appropriately when learning about a family crisis than does the family. Often this is because so much is happening to them that they cannot put the energy into anything else. This does not mean they are not concerned or that they don't care. It simply means they are willing to let others take care of matters. They are extremely grateful that people (particularly their family) have been honest enough with them to trust them and that they will keep them informed as an active member of the family. It also makes them feel that people will be honest with them about their own situation. Whatever the crisis, it usually cannot be kept a secret forever. The patient will find out even if everything ends up being perfect. Someday something will come up, something will be said, and the truth will have to be known. And that is when the patient asks, "Why didn't you tell me the truth?" "What else didn't you tell me?" "How do I know you'll tell me the truth in the future?" "How much does what I think mean if you don't tell me things as important as my wife's heart attack?"

Unfortunately, things do not always "just get better." The crisis can get worse. As I have already said, it is much easier to cope with situations as they are evolving than at the end of the line—especially if lies and cover-ups have been used from the beginning. In the situation I have been relating to you, the patient's wife had an extension of the heart damage a few days later and died suddenly in the hospital. Her initial heart attack was at night, and we (the family and I) told the patient the following morning. (I actually had to do the talking. It is extremely difficult for family who are so close to the event to tell the patient. It hurts too much—which is part of the reason they don't want the patient told. I can do the work for them. They need to be here so that all hear it together. They can cry; they can retell it and give the details. Then I can help guide them with what to do next. What is important is that everyone knows what everyone else knows.) The patient's surgery, which was scheduled for the next day, was put on hold. The patient had very critical obstructions, and we advised him not to leave the hospital. Instead, we arranged for the patient and his wife to talk by phone, to say what they had to say to each other and decide how and when to proceed with the patient's surgery. The wife was stable, but we discussed the possibilities of complications. The patient was not safe without surgery. They decided together that the patient should go ahead with surgery as scheduled. During his operation I stayed in touch with the coronary intensive care unit where his wife was so that she knew how he was doing. The patient did well and went to his room on his second day after surgery. His wife continued to recover well and was also moved to a regular hospital room. They talked again by phone. The following day she died. While part of the family was with her, I told the patient with his son. We cried, retold the details, and discussed what was to be done next. The patient and family grieved together. They kept him informed of all the events, and he continued to recover without complication. Death is never easy for those who are left behind, but there doesn't have to be any regrets. We don't have control of everything, and reality is reality. If it is dealt with honestly, humanly, those who remain behind can live a life that is good, though forever different.

There are other situations, much less vital, that cause a great deal of distress and concern for the family. One that people are least prepared for and find most disconcerting is when a patient is confused and disoriented. We do a great deal to interfere with a person's unique makeup when he or she undergoes open heart surgery. There is nothing normal about having your chest opened, about someone handling your heart while machines breathe for you and circulate your blood. Then you're made to take back the work of pumping the blood around and get your chest closed up with all kinds of tubes hanging out. Then you're taken to the intensive care unit, where there is no semblance of a normal life style. You are not permitted to have any control over anything, not even your breathing, for some hours. You have nothing to say (literally—you can't talk with the breathing tube in) about anything that is done to you, how it is done, or when it is done. You get strange medications you're not used to, you don't get to eat or go to the bathroom, you don't have any idea whether it is day or night, and, what's even worse, you're not allowed to sleep and you're not allowed to stay awake! It makes one wonder why every patient isn't "crazy"! As a rule, patients do very well because they have been briefed as to what to expect: Their recall of the first twenty-four hours or so after surgery isn't very good, but by that time they have regained some controls and leave the intensive care unit a short time later. Some patients seem to have more trouble than others: (1) those who may have disease in the vessels supplying the brain or other physiologic process altering brain function; (2) those done as an emergency without any explanation about what is happening, or briefing as to what to expect and no time to get used to the idea; (3) those who have a complicated course with a long intensive care stay; (4) those who normally are very assertive and aggressive in controlling their lives and others, are used to telling others what to do and having it done their way, and are competitive and time-oriented; and (5) those who have little or no symptoms and have not been ill with their disease.

Patients who have a "post-op psychosis"—such as confusion, disorientation, belligerence, paranoia, hallucinations, and the like—believe everything they think and feel. These beliefs usually center around conspiracies, torture, imprisonment or concentration camps, punishment, and sexual assaults and abuse. Whatever the case may be, patients see themselves as responding normally to an abnormal situation. Such patients may (and often do) say hurtful things to their family and act in an unbecoming manner. In fact, families often feel that the patient is not the same person as before the surgery, and, indeed, the patient is not. But the condition is temporary. Patients recover from this experience, usually without residual effects. They may never even remember any of it. Families remember everything; patients remember only what was true for them—which may have nothing to do with reality. An example is the patient who refuses to see or talk to anyone in his family and is angry at all the hospital staff—especially the nurses and doctors. He believes he is being tortured, while just outside the door his family is having a party. He feels his family is letting him suffer at the hands of these people while they are having a good time.

I have learned that there is nothing that you can do to try to convince the patient otherwise. The patient truly believes that what he or she thinks is happening is reality. Though these delusions should not be reinforced, the patient needs to know that you accept the fact that he or she believes them. Even years later, when patients can say intellectually that they know that what they thought couldn't have been true, they nevertheless recall it that way. For them the events will never change. That was the way they experienced it, and that is OK; it doesn't have to change.

The family usually needs a great deal of help with all of that. They need support to hang in there. The episodes are time-limited. Patients usually get better as they recover—as they get less medication and gain more control in a more normal life-style setting.

To summarize, I want to leave you with four main thoughts. (1) Heart surgery is a big deal. Often there are many more facets to it than are initially considered by the patient or family. (2) People can never know for sure how they will respond to a situation until they are in the midst of it. Most people need assistance when they are in a new situation that is threatening and very close to them. They need help to cope in the manner that is most effective for them and will leave them in the best state of health. (3) The big thing is not to panic. You can't change history. Facts are facts, and they can be dealt with realistically. It's a case of sorting out what the alternatives are and utilizing every situation for the benefits that can be gained from it. We only take this trip that is life once. We need to enjoy it and make every minute the best it can be without looking back. (4) People need people to get safely through difficult times. That is what it is all about, and that is what makes it all worthwhile.

Mrs. Nadler's deep compassion for humanity needs no amplification by me. This chapter would rightly be complete with her last written word, as there is nothing more to add. However, there is a special anecdote that belongs here.

On the very day that Mrs. Nadler went into labor to give birth to her daughter, her sense of commitment was so strong that she spent the day at the clinic working, even though she was having labor pains. Two weeks to the day after the baby was born, she resumed her counseling activities.

Furthermore, during the latter days of the pregnancy, the approaching birth, the promise of a new life, seemed to carry its own special message to those who were close to death.

11

POSTOPERATIVE CARE

The Cocktail Party.
The Patients
on Floor Seven

You didn't really believe all that stuff about wild parties and dancing girls, did you? Well, some of it is true, as you shall see.

Unit 7Q really does have a cocktail party every night at 8:30. But that first night was hardly the time to appreciate frivolities. I was just too tired to do much more than raise my head. I probably slept right through the first party and never even heard it.

You see, when you get to your room in the wheelchair, you're too weak to move more than two or three steps. They support you as you get out of the chair, and they ease you into a clean, comfortable-looking bed, where you're going to get lots of sleep and rest.

You can eat sitting up or lying down, and your mood is one of exuberance. You feel like saying—to no one in particular, except maybe to yourself—"I made it!" Your voice quivers and quakes when you talk, and when you look your body over and see all the holes and incisions, you marvel at the resilience of the human body—and yours in particular.

When I was wheeled into the room, I noticed that I again had a roommate. Like the others, he had the bed next to the window. His wife was in the room, and he was already moving about fairly well, although he still walked with a stiff, hesitant gait, his eyes glued to the floor. His operation had been about three days before mine. This time I was in a more forgiving mood, and in fact I was happy to have a roommate. I figured if I needed help in a hurry, I had someone close by to help out or get attention. His presence was a source of comfort. I even smiled at his wife. I was happy to have all the friends I could get.

This fellow had an interesting history. He was an executive at General Motors. He lived in Detroit, and his wife was staying at the Clinic Inn. She had driven down and was waiting to drive him back home when they released him. Like

147

myself, he had been through this operation once before. But in his case it only lasted a year. He was remarkably cheerful for it all, and when I first encountered him, he was already strolling the halls and telling jokes. His home had just been sold (while he was in the hospital), and he and his wife were planning to move within thirty days to Florida. He was retiring. I couldn't help but admire his pluckiness and confidence in the future and his keen wit.

On the day before he was scheduled to go home, he happened to glance at his wrist bracelet and discovered it had the wrong name on it. Actually it was discovered by the nurse, who checked his name before giving him medication. These bracelets, which are installed by the hospital on the day you arrive, are used to identify you throughout your blackout stages. When they put one on your wrist, you are asked to verify that the name on the tag is yours. Hence, it is hard to see how anyone could end up with the wrong bracelet. He admitted checking it at the time, so somewhere in between day one and recovery, he had apparently lost the original and acquired a new one. Sometimes nurses cut them off to make room for an IV, and put a new ID bracelet on the other wrist.

I kidded him at the time and told him they had probably given him the wrong operation and that the other fellow got his. The nurse, horrified at my remark, said, "Don't even suggest that!" but my roommate laughed nervously. He insisted he had gotten the right operation because it was the right bracelet when he went into surgery. Besides, he had also met his surgeon several times, as I had mine. I immediately checked my own bracelet uneasily, to be sure I was properly identified. There have been errors of this type that have resulted in serious problems. Some patients have gotten the wrong medication, some the wrong operation. I read about a patient that had a kidney removed by mistake. I am not aware of any of these things having happened at the clinic, but it is clear that both the patient and the staff must work together to avoid mistakes. Nurses are usually required, for example, to verify directly with the patient any medicines that are to be administered.

My roommate had a long drive home to Detroit, about 200 miles. That seemed like an awfully long trip to me. I didn't envy him. After my first operation, I recalled that my drive home—of just a few miles—was very unsettling. It was raining; the roads were slippery, and my wife seemed to be unusually heavy-footed. The speedometer reached fifty several times, and I agonized over the possibility of an accident. I could see my chest popping open like a ruptured watermelon, with seeds and red meat splattered everywhere. I asked her to slow down, but she just seemed to go faster. Every bump was like a California earthquake. The ride was a sheer nightmare. My chest stayed together, no thanks to my imagination.

My second ride home, this time from the clinic, over a much greater distance and in snowy weather, proved to be almost carefree. Prior to leaving the clinic, I had discussed my earlier experiences and fears with my wife and had secured her promise to drive with sanity. By this, I meant not more than fifty on the interstate going home. She did exactly this, but I felt so confident on the way home that I became impatient with her puttering driving. How the times, and my attitudes, had changed from one operation to another! What had happened to those old fears and uncertainties that had plagued me the first time? Why was I so much more self-assured this time? I do not know how my roommate fared on his trip home, but his confidence suggested he did well. How lucky are those who die but one death!

My roommate set a standard for me in other respects as well.

On my second day in Unit 7Q, they pulled out the neck IV, removed the nose tubes providing oxygen, and started letting me go to the bathroom. I was rid of the bedpan, thank heavens!

Then I was allowed, and encouraged, to walk the halls. One complete cycle around the nurse's station, the elevators, and the central area, they told me pointedly, was a tenth of a mile. Ten trips was a mile. My partner was already up to ten trips. He worked at it diligently. Every time I saw him, he was shuffling up and down the hallway.

"Don't overdo it when you first start," they had also said. So I walked out into the hall fifty feet and nearly collapsed. My heart pounded, my knees wobbled, and I wanted to sit down. There was no place to sit, the nearest chair was thirty feet away, and I didn't think I could make it back to the security and safety of my bed. So I stood and waited and finally got back, my heart pounding madly. I lay down and rested, listening to my pounding heart.

"You did real good!" my roommate said with pride. He was glad to be rooming with someone as tough as I. I could see it in his eyes. I couldn't read his mind, however, and he was a super salesman. Since I couldn't let him down, I managed to make a second trip again later that day. I even included a trip to the bathroom. I felt all drained out, and my heart seemed to be pleading with me to give it a rest, but I pretended to smile.

By the time he left, a few days later, I was up to two laps around the "track." He was now doing twenty.

As I ranged the halls, I ran into my old roommates from before the operation. They were walking, too. They looked tired and weary, like characters from a zombie movie who had had their brains removed. All motions were mechanical shuffles. Their faces were serious and emotionless as they concentrated on getting one foot ahead of the other, in painfully precise slow-motion. When we met, we didn't talk. We didn't smile. We just stood and looked at each other. A word or two was spoken, but we were too tired and weak to really communicate. We were too anxious to get back to port and lie down. We were all battle-weary.

About halfway through the week, they called my name on the P.A. system, along with about twelve others, and told us to assemble in the hallway at the nurse's station. I took my time getting out of bed, and when I finally appeared outside my door, in my slow-motion shuffle, I looked about for an army drill sergeant. Instead I was met by a good-looking nurse who told me I was going to class. Gathering in the hall were my cohorts, many of whom had their wives or children with them. "Class?" I wondered. "How about next week?" But the nurse insisted, so I fell in.

"Class" was on the next floor, so we had to walk to the elevator, crowd in as a group, and take a short ride. A technician met us and guided us to the classroom.

The room was set up like a schoolroom with a lectern and blackboard. There were about twenty individual folding chairs in the room.

Both the patients and the families attended this class. This was a postoperative session to prepare for life beyond the hospital.

Here you are told about the need to walk every day, working up slowly until you can cover four or five miles. Since it was winter, the technician suggested using a public mall.

Various problems and experiences were discussed, such as wearing surgical stockings to reduce the swelling in your legs from the incisions. You are told that you can drive a car in three weeks and that a checkup will be scheduled with your doctor for six weeks hence. Those who lived nearby usually came to the clinic to see their doctor; the others saw their doctor at home.

The session lasted about an hour. In the midst of it, one of the patients suddenly went limp, his eyes rolled, and he fell out of his chair onto the floor. (Fainting is not an uncommon thing for those who are in a weakened condition, and even for those in the best of health. In the Navy on the drill-field in summer, for example, I saw over thirty sailors pass out while standing at attention during a review. For the group at the class, however, it was more frightening than it should have been, no doubt because of our timidity with respect to our own selves.)

The effect on the group was electric. Terror swept the room. Even the visitors were unable to react effectively. As we watched in horror, a couple of nurses began ministering to the poor man. He just lay there like blubber, his mouth open and his eyes distended. The technician told us to leave the room. He guided us to another room, where we waited, quivering from weakness, still standing but badly in need of support. The room was hushed; everyone was afraid to talk.

Suddenly, one of the patients spoke up in a commanding voice. "There's nothing to fear. This happens all the time. Just relax and you'll be all right."

I looked at him, and he seemed to be speaking from experience. One of the patients muttered, "He must be a doctor from the clinic who just had an operation." The rumor spread, and the tension in the room began to dissipate. No one smiled, but as the fears diminished, a few began to talk.

The man who had counseled the group was a big man

with a totally bald head who looked like a stocky Telly Savalas or, more precisely—for those who are old enough to remember—like Erich Von Stroheim. He was not the type whose word you would normally question.

It turned out, when I met him later at a cocktail party and had a chance to talk to him, that he was not a doctor at all. He was a tire salesman from Akron. He had learned his gift of command from the Army. He had been a field sergeant and had seen many comrades die in action. He had learned, then, the need for someone to calm the panic among the others. He had merely carried this gift over into the present situation, much to the relief of all of us. This same man is the patient I mentioned earlier who had had the heart-valve operation, who had contracted pneumonia and almost died the day before he was to be operated on. He was now as strong and able as any of us and was feeling excellent for the time that had elapsed. His performance at the training program had been superb, and being a good actor he could have been elected president that day. He certainly was a hero to everyone.

After a few minutes of waiting around, the group was ushered back to the training room. We were all eager to get back to our rooms and lie down. We didn't want a repeat performance like the one we'd just witnessed.

The technician advised us that the patient had just passed out and was now doing fine. This helped, but it didn't eliminate the uneasiness completely. When we finally traipsed back to the elevator and returned "home," it was great to get back.

The situation is a disturbing and embarassing example of the frailty of human compassion under stressed conditions. Had the man passed out under other circumstances, when we were fully recovered, any one of us would have jumped in to help; but being terribly weak and almost totally dependent, we thought only of ourselves. Only one man among us had the courage to rise above his own needs and care for the others. I wish I could tell you this man's name. I tried to find him later, but it was too late. To me, he was a real hero and I hope that he reads this book.

I might mention here the almost total absence of women patients in the group. Out of about thirty patients in 7Q, there were only two women. One of these women was in her late eighties. She was very weak and walked the halls only with the aid of a nurse at her side. But despite her age, she did remarkably well. She was an exceedingly cheerful person and seemed to enjoy the attention she was getting. The other woman was in her seventies. The average age of the male patients was between fifty and fifty-five. There is no doubt that the good Lord has seen fit to discriminate against the men in this type of operation. Furthermore, Congress has done nothing to correct this condition, and the courts have been completely silent on the issue.

The preponderance of men at the time led me to suspect that this was not an accident. I resolved to corroborate the facts on a return visit several months later. At this time, I was able to obtain a more accurate count, thanks to the help of the nurse in charge.

We found that in both wards on the seventh floor, there were sixteen women and sixty men—a total of seventy-six patients under cardiovascular care. Of the eight women whose ages we checked, three were in their seventies. We also checked the ages of eight of the men. The oldest was sixty-six; the average was in the early fifties. I can also add the ages of two close friends who had the operation: They were fifty-three and forty-five. My own age was fifty-one at the time of the first operation and fifty-seven at the time of the second. Hence, men seem to have the operation at a younger age, and more men are involved than women.

Better methods of detection of the disease are having the effect of catching people at a younger age than was the case a few years ago. In addition, older people who were once considered ineligible for the operation are now being operated on with considerable success. A few years ago, these same people might have died from the operation.

Hence, the age span of patients who have open heart surgery at the clinic is widening over time, as the operation and techniques of detection keep improving, and the statistics I have quoted are changing.

Women are still clearly in the minority, but as more women are engaged in higher-stress job situations, more women are having heart problems at a younger age, unfortunately. Hopefully they will have greater success in dealing with stress than men. My own belief is that they will.

My findings, and my imprecise survey, are also supported by the experiences at Akron, where only a few women were in the cardiac care units during my tenure.

My discovery of this imbalance in nature disturbed me less for its injustice than its effect upon my long-planned entry into the cocktail party. Imagine a cocktail party with only two women and all those men!

And now having mentioned it, I cannot keep you in suspense any longer. Let's go to the cocktail party.

My first cocktail party came about the third night after my operation. I was in bed, as usual, when I heard the call come over the P.A. system. It came at 8 P.M. and was given in the mellifluous tones of a sultry female nurse. "Everyone out of their rooms for the cocktail party." I wanted to jump right out of bed and go, but I was too tired. I resolved to go the next time.

The next night the call came again. In ludicrous anticipation, I forced myself upright, put my slippers on, and bumbled my way out the door into the hallway. The party was just outside my door. I couldn't have gone one step further. I didn't have the strength. Anticipation alone kept me going. A ring of empty chairs and tables surrounded a bowl of ginger ale and a setup of cookies. Three or four hedonism-bent patients shuffled out of their rooms and hurried down the hall in slow-motion. They were gradually joined by others of equal mettle. Our bald-headed field sergeant was there, plus my old roommates and the two women I mentioned.

I had endured as long as I could. The cookies didn't look good. The ginger ale didn't look good. I was too weak to sit up and talk. I turned and went back to bed. I fell asleep instantly. It had been a tiring party.

A day or two later, I stayed long enough to play chess with another patient. He was two days ahead of me, and he cheated. He outlasted me. He won, I consoled myself, because I was too weak in the end to outlast him. Chess is such a grueling game, and he had taken advantage of me.

As Christmas approached, the halls and rooms began to empty out. By Christmas Eve, the ward, which had held about thirty-five patients, was down to a mere handful. The operating schedule dropped off from seventeen patients per day to six or less. Only extreme emergency cases were going through now.

The parties continued at the same furious pace, however, but they had lost their zip. Instead of twenty persons sitting around in a circle, barely talking, we now had only two or three. Our voices still quivered when we talked, and it was hard to say much without tiring. It was easier to socialize by sitting quietly in an overstuffed chair, looking at the floor. A grunt or two would keep the party going indefinitely. As we got stronger, we discussed things like where we came from and what we did, using short sentences so we could be sure of finishing them before our strength gave out. The patients ready to go home in a day or two were naturally the most chipper and talkative. But by Christmas Eve we had lost them and were forced to scrape the bottom of the barrel for our entertainment. I became one of the chief entertainers because I was stronger than almost anybody else. I challenged a great big guy to a fight, and he only grinned. He knew I was better than him.

The nurses did an admirable job of dispensing cheer; with the approach of Christmas, and the constant reminder of music on the radio, they had a difficult job. It was sad to watch the others go, while you stayed behind.

There was no great amount of pain. Mostly soreness and numbness. Two aspirin would last for four hours. A couple of pain pills a day was usually enough.

My family showed up daily, and I was always glad to see them, so I practiced being grouchy with them. That way I could share the suffering with them. There was no reason they should be having fun when I wasn't. They hadn't gone through all this pain and suffering, so why should they be happy? They always walked in with big smiles on their faces, but I got rid of those in a hurry. Grouchiness, I found, was a great equalizer. Before long we were all growling at each other. When they left, I was glad to see them go, because I couldn't stand all those cranks in the room with me. When they were gone it was always sad and lonely. You can love your family and still not be as good to them as you'd like.

From the day of my operation until after I had been home for a few days, I found myself constantly covered with sweat. (My wife tells me that horses *sweat*, men *perspire*, and women *glow*. But to me, that clammy, wet feeling was sweat.) When I woke up at night, the bed was wet. It was quite embarrassing at first, until I found out the cause. I was running a slight temperature from the operation, the nurse told me. I guess this is common for people who have been operated on.

My first days at home, I lay on the couch in the family room, near the fireplace, and my wife kept asking me if I wanted a fire. She couldn't understand why I turned her down. She insisted that I ought to be cold.

This was a far cry from my first days in the hospital, when I almost froze to death. My roommate with the bad-shaving experience had the same problem. The nurse blamed our problem on our poor circulation, but we suspected the hospital hadn't paid the heat bill.

We called the maintenance man in to check the thermostat, and he insisted that it agreed with his pocket thermometer. It was obvious that he didn't know what he was talking about. I had only to listen to my chattering teeth to know that. My roommate nodded in disgust. So we devised a method for cheating the system.

Now what I'm about to tell you is highly classified and should not be revealed to just anybody. It is worth the price of the book itself, so if you've been feeling cheated up until now—which you probably have—please let your resentment go no further.

My friend, who had a little larceny in his heart, plus a desire to keep warm as well, was caught tampering with the thermostat. Now, hospitals—and most public offices—know that there are people like him in every room, so they fix the thermostat so it can't be adjusted. But my friend discovered a devious way to fool the thermostat. He did this by putting wet paper towels over it to cool it down. At first I wondered what he was up to, until I caught him in the act. I had put wet cloths on my children's heads when they were sick with a fever, but I'd never seen it done to a sick thermostat. The idea struck me as fiendishly clever. It met with my hearty approval. We became instant accomplices.

The system worked marvelously. The room heated right up and stayed there until the towel dried out. Between him and me, we managed to keep the towel wet all day and night. We even took turns getting up at night to douse the thermostat.

Our problem was the nurses. They couldn't be trusted. They complained of the heat every time they came into the room. They claimed it felt like a boiler room. Some of those evil nurses even removed the towel and scolded us. "That's a no-no," they said, shaking a finger at us. My partner looked at me and shrugged. "They're not paying the bill," he seemed to say, to which I nodded my full approval. Then, as soon as the nurse left the room, we reinvested the thermostat with its damp cover.

Once I had the operation, as I said, this was no problem. I supplied my own heat. The hospital didn't have to pay the added heat bill. So they could now take the difference off my bill, which I'm sure they did.

This wetting-down-the-thermostat trick can be carried over to hotels and public offices where the thermostats never seem to be set right. Everybody in this world seems to be determined to freeze cardiovascular patients to death. It offers all kinds of potential for those of us with cold hearts and cold feet. I don't need it all the time anymore, fortunately, because I keep warm pretty well, thanks to my operation. But there are those out there who do and who can profit by this knowledge.

Dr. Sheldon stopped in regularly and checked me out. On the day before Christmas he commented on my progress. "If you keep progressing like this," he said, "maybe you can go home in a day or two." I nodded my head, but I didn't believe him. I expected to be there several days longer. I told my wife not to plan on my being home the next day. In fact, I told her not to come up until the afternoon, so she could spend Christmas morning with the family.

But Dr. Sheldon showed up early Christmas Day, checked me out, and released me to go home. I called my wife and told her to come and get me, and forget about the family.

I was still wired for a heart pacemaker, so they sent for a technician to remove the wires. She removed the stitches holding the wires in place in my chest and then pulled lightly on each wire. This caused a small twinge of pain—no more than a pin prick. I wanted to scream in agony but bravely held back as she gently tugged at the wire. All the time, she kept saying, "Are you OK? Are you OK? Let me know if it hurts." Then the wire slid out of the small hole in my chest. When she came to a wire that was stubborn and wouldn't come loose from its implantation in the surface of the heart muscle, she just clipped it off with wire cutters and left it there inside my chest.

When it was all over, and the sweat—excuse me, perspiration—was pouring off my forehead, she looked at me and said, "There. That wasn't so bad, was it?"

I nodded to her. She was very pretty, and I couldn't tell her the truth, so I smiled bravely and said, "No, I rather enjoyed it!" Then she told me they would keep an eye on me for a couple of hours to make sure my heart hadn't started to act up and that my pulse was steady.

After a few more checkups, I got dressed and was waiting, ready to go, when my wife arrived.

The man in uniform I told you about met me in the hallway with a wheelchair, and I was on my way. This time I didn't mind the ride, even though I could almost have walked it. By now I was a professional wheelchair rider, sitting tall in the saddle, a pleasant smile on my face. As people looked at me, they smiled back. They knew I was going home. The nurses on floor seven were the happiest of all.

12

GOING
HOME

*Christmas Day.
Recovery at Home*

Christmas Day! What a wonderful time to be going home. When we drove into the driveway, the snow was falling lightly and the sun was shining. On the front of the garage, completely spanning the wide door, was a large paper sign emblazoned with the words "Welcome Home, Dad!" As we opened the car door and got out, the front door burst open and Carol and Nick came out to welcome me. Our dog Tigger ran out and jumped up on me, whimpering and wagging her body. Unlike most dogs, her tail doesn't work separately. Tigger—whom we called a Tasmanian lop-ear to establish her credentials in the neighborhood—was an import from the dog pound and a member of the family.

I walked into the house. It smelled good and familiar. The Christmas tree, sitting in front of the large window in the living room, was covered with decorations and lights. Under the tree were a number of presents, gaily wrapped and carefully placed at random.

My wife had the family room prepared for my arrival. A blanket and pillow lay on the couch. Wood was stacked in the fireplace, awaiting a match.

As I lay down, my wife prepared the first home-cooked meal that I'd had for days. It was little more than toast and fruit, but it was a banquet.

My married daughters Kathleen and Jacquie and their husbands Bob and Mark arrived. My grandson Harley stood by, uncertain of his place.

Everyone exchanged presents and talked happily, while I kept to myself on the couch.

The next day a few visitors arrived. My wife did a marvelous job of scheduling friends and relatives throughout the week to avoid overtaxing me and wearing me out. On Christmas Day, the phone rang intermittently with calls from friends and relatives. People whom I hadn't seen for years called and talked to Ginny to offer their best wishes. Some friends sent flowers. Many sent cards.

Few people in this world have been as lucky and happy as I that day. I had no regrets at leaving the hospital, no concerns for my well-being that I couldn't get right at home.

This comes in contrast to some of my earlier experiences and the experiences of many others when they first come home. For some it is not at all unusual to feel apprehensive and depressed on leaving the hospital. Sometimes those feelings are prompted by concern about leaving the security provided by a team of medical experts supported by elaborate equipment, as opposed to the home remedies that lie ahead.

We tend to forget or minimize the benefits that home care offers. We tend to forget that *we can get well at home, too!* And, further, that help, if needed, is as close as the telephone. We have difficulty in some cases realizing that the doctors would not be sending us home unless they felt it wise and beneficial to do so. This is their business. They are the experts.

Notwithstanding this fact, on my trip home following the first operation, I was beset with a number of strange fears that have been noticeably absent this time.

I mentioned the fear of riding in the car as my wife drove home. This time these fears were totally absent, and the ride home was pleasant and relaxed.

For a long time after the first operation, being in crowds was very upsetting. Elevators made me feel panicky. When the door would close, I felt myself wanting to get out into the open air. I was afraid of being trapped, cooped up, unable to fend for myself. I dreaded travel. I was afraid I would lose my strength and wouldn't get back. There were constant fears of becoming helpless and unable to manage for myself.

None of these fears was rational, but they affected my life for several years. I learned to live with them, but they influenced my decisions. I have already mentioned their effect on my business and financial life.

By a strange contrast, I have had none of these uncertainties this time. My confidence has been greater this time than at any time since my problems began.

If I had any fears this last time, it was that I would not get home on schedule. I was eager to be discharged. Instead of excuses for staying and emphasizing imaginary problems, as patients sometimes do, I was concerned that something would crop up unexpectedly that would keep me longer. I had fluid in my lungs at the time of my discharge, for example. They knew about it. I suspected it, but they sent me home anyway. Fluid is fairly common with surgical patients. It takes time to clear up and can be monitored by outpatient x-rays and during the periodic checkups. I didn't know this at the time, so naturally it was of some concern.

Other than these "borrowing trouble" type of worries, however, the old crop of fears had completely vanished, so that I entered the world as a renewed individual with a great deal of vigor and confidence.

The before-and-after difference is evident from a pair of experiences. Four or five months after the first operation, I took a trip to Texas. (This is the trip mentioned by Dr. Ormond in chapter 4.) The weather was marvelous, and I did my walking outside. I only worked two hours a day and relaxed at the Hotel. But I came down with severe chest pains and was hospitalized.

Three months after the second operation, I went to New York and New Jersey on business. While there, we had one of the worst blizzards on record. Over twelve inches of snow fell on New York City. Airports were closed everywhere. Cars could scarcely travel. To get from my motel to the plant I was visiting, a distance of two miles, it took over two hours by car.

Earlier, I would have been beside myself with fear and anxiety. But not this time. I felt relaxed. There was no apprehension. I had no irresistible urge to rush for home and safety. Somewhere between operation one and operation two, I had regained my balance and perspective on life.

I may also have been better off physically, but I think the big difference was mental attitude. (The attitude on the flight up, by the way, bothered me some, but returning and in subsequent flights that has not been a problem.)

There are many benefits, of course, to getting away from the hospital. Your spouse and family make excellent nurses, because they give you far more attention than you deserve. It is better than you ever got the last few days in the hospital. Instead of that miserable, bland hospital food, you now get everything you want—even pheasant under glass, if you should so desire. They run and get your slippers or your housecoat. If you have left anything upstairs, they run up and get it to save you the trip. They're more afraid of the stairs than you are. When you climb the stairs, you pant and pull on the railing and work your way up. At the top, you catch your breath and wait for your strength to return. Your knees are always the weakest part. They turn to rubber at the slightest provocation. You can feel the strength drain out and then back in as you wait. The result is far more frightening to the observer than to the patient.

This is the perfect moment of your life, and you must be prepared to take advantage of it. You may pass this way only once, and it shouldn't be spoiled by feelings of guilt or human tendencies.

This special catering, for me, actually began while I was still in the hospital.

As you know, you get to order anything you want from a menu they bring you to fill in each day. At first I ordered only a few things. I had no appetite for a lot of food. When it came, I had no taste for what I ordered, and much of it was returned. Worse yet, the nurses or kitchen staff kept a record of what I ate. Since I didn't want to end up on an IV, I stuffed something down. The combination of lack of appetite (making all food taste like starch) and apparently tasteless cooking were almost insurmountable obstacles. I solved my problem in two ways: I ordered a little of everything, so I could taste and choose the things that tasted best, and I had my wife bring in a few things that sounded good. I was not on any particular diet at the time, so getting energy was my first concern. Unfortunately, the food my wife brought in tasted no better than the hospital food. The problem was me, not the food.

Gradually I began to eat better and was almost up to the intake of a small child when I headed home.

My stomach gave me trouble the last couple of days at the hospital and continued to plague me for about two weeks at home. I finally asked Dr. Moats for something, and from then on my appetite blossomed—too much, in fact, because I began gaining weight. It would be an ill wind that didn't blow some good, and even the bypass operation has its special blessings. Having gone through it twice, I have found that it is consistently good for a loss of nineteen pounds. This beats any Hollywood diet or other touted weight-loss plan by a mile. It's an almost guaranteed result, and you get it free. As a side benefit, you get rid of the angina and other chest pains that were bothering you.

My sixth-week visit to Dr. Sheldon came along at about this time, and it sticks in my mind with clarity for a couple of reasons (of which dieting was one).

Dr. Sheldon has developed a very effective method for handling these checkups: He has his nurse give you an in-depth interview and physical checkup that lasts about forty-five minutes. The nurse follows a detailed routine and discusses your experiences since leaving the hospital carefully, taking notes as she goes. When she is through, Dr. Sheldon ushers you into his office. He rechecks some of the physical tests she has made and then discusses with you each point on the nurse's questionnaire. He also reviews your personal history, which was prepared during your stay at the clinic. The result is an extremely effective and complete analysis and interview. I was impressed, as you can see, my earlier remarks on visits to doctors notwithstanding.

During the course of the interview, one of the questions that came up had to do with my appetite. I told him it was getting too good and that my weight had stabilized at 152, which was the weight I would like to maintain. He grinned and said, "As your appetite builds up, you'll gain a few pounds."

He was right, of course. I had to start watching my weight almost at once. To top it off, in April, less than four months after the operation, my wife, daughter Carol, Nick, and I took an eleven-day cruise to the Caribbean. We sailed on the *Rotterdam*, a Dutch ship, and hit four islands; but mostly we ate. My wife described the trip later as having "wall-to-wall food." The food on board was fabulous. Every evening meal was eleven courses, with a wide choice of selections, and of a quality equal to the best of restaurants. Food was served from 7 in the morning until 9:30 at night. There was a midnight buffet and an afternoon tea. In addition, food was available in some part of the ship twenty-four hours a day. By the third or fourth day

I was forced to cut back or turn into a blimp. I walked the deck faithfully every day for an hour, one complete lap being 950 feet. I had lots of company from joggers and other walkers. I played golf for an hour on the driving range. And I gained five pounds.

Since I had resolved to keep my weight to 154, the day I got back I went on a diet. It was much harder getting it off than putting it on, but as I write this, three weeks later, I have returned to my weight of 152. If I seem smug, it's because I have developed the perfect system for dieting. This, too, I will pass on free of charge.

You must, of course, check with your doctor and lawyer before you embark on any diet: the former to make sure it's safe, and the latter to find out how much your estate can collect if you die. From what I can gather, diets are more deadly than open heart operations. Hence, you may want to forgo dieting and get a bypass instead. But if you're really serious about losing weight by willpower, here's the plan.

You've got to quit eating so much! I did it by setting a reasonable goal of a couple of hundred calories less than my normal intake. As I ate each thing, I looked up the calories and posted the number on a tally sheet. I kept a running total, and when the sum was equal to my goal, I quit.

I didn't quit keeping the record. I quit eating. From that time on, I ate only celery and carrots, which don't count, until I went to bed. Presto! In twenty-some days I was back to my former trim and slim weight. Now, if it creeps up again, and I lose my willpower, my only recourse is another bypass or getting fat. But this one time, my diet was a great success, and I'm pleased to pass my system along. I only hope you will keep it secret until I can write a book on it.

When you're in the hospital, you'll find that your doctor, the dietitian, or the nursing staff can advise you properly on how to modify your eating habits. Naturally, it is wise to reduce coronary risk factors as much as possible by reducing salt, cholesterol, and saturated fats in the diet. It also is important to keep an appropriate weight for your height—that is, to avoid being overweight *or* underweight. Moderation and common sense usually are the best guides in both eating and drinking.

These things are easy to say but very hard to live by. Like smoking, we all know the rules and agree with the need to observe them, but we keep on breaking the laws of nature anyway. Between my first and second operation, a period of six years, my weight gain was less than two pounds per year. That's a pretty sneaky increase to have to live with. You can't even see yourself getting fatter. Unlike cigarette smoking, which you can give up completely (with any luck), with eating you're stuck. You've got to eat every day to keep alive, and as a result you're called upon daily to exercise restraint. As a result, I found it easier to give up smoking than to give up my daily orgy of food.

The cruise was kind of a sop to my ego and a peace offering to my wife. There came a time when my family began to suspect that I was taking advantage of them. I seemed to be spending entirely too much time lying on the couch, demanding attention. About the time they began catching me doing for myself when they were out of the room, they started clamping down. As the clamor mounted, I had to repay them in kind, so we took a cruise. The fact that we were going to escape from Ohio's nasty April weather, with its snow, sleet, and cold rain, had nothing to do with it.

I began working the week I got home from the hospital. Work at that time amounted to a few phone calls. Later I added a trip to a plant to do some work for my firm. My first visit lasted only a few minutes, and by the time I was allowed to drive, I had visited the plant twice to check on progress for our project.

On January 9, a close friend and client flew in from New Jersey to cover a project we were doing for his company. He came by invitation and stayed overnight at my home. We went out to dinner that evening and generally the dinner went very well. But when I got home, I discovered I wasn't as strong as I had thought.

I became very weak and went to bed almost as soon as I arrived. My heart began to race and slow down in cycles. It beat like a drum in my ears. I couldn't relax, and I felt like I was teetering on the edge of a cliff, about to plunge over. This panicky tension lasted almost all night. I called Dr. Grow (at 3 o'clock in the morning) and described my symptoms. His first reaction was to put me in the hospital. I had hesitated about calling him for this reason, and, at my urging, he finally agreed to see how I did during the night. I had drunk two cups of coffee at dinner and a Coke at home; my normal intake was less than a cup of coffee a week. It was almost certain that my problem was caffeine-induced and that I was suffering from over-stimulation caused by my weakened condition and lack of practice.

By morning I felt better, but not much better. Even that next night I was still charged up and had trouble sleeping. For the next two days I spent more time prone than upright. My body felt weak and washed out and nervous. When the phone rang, my whole body jumped.

My friend beat a hasty exit the next morning, believing he had been the cause of my problem. He wasn't, of course. Had I been less incautious and less excited by my first night out, I am sure this would never have happened.

At very little encouragement from Dr. Grow, I kept away from coffee and cola for several weeks.

This weakness that plagues the heart patient, of which I have spoken also in climbing the stairs, is less a result of the heart operation or heart damage than a function of inactivity. The muscles atrophy from disuse. Even a healthy college student who spends a week in bed loses almost 15 percent of his muscular strength. It should be no surprise, then, that after virtually weeks of inactivity, spread out on a cot or bed in your home or the hospital, you have become prone to being tired and feeling weak. Your strength can only be regained by a program of exercise. Walking is an especially good exercise after coronary bypass graft surgery, but it should be done with moderation.

Many patients who leave the hospital go through a traumatic period of depression. There is an emotional letdown after the operation that may cause these feelings. Progress may not seem fast enough. You may be anxious to do more. Sometimes there are temporary setbacks and relapses that are disturbing. Time may seem to stand still.

Sometimes talking it over with a close member of the family helps. Family members themselves may unknowingly bring on depression.

Some things are a constant source of irritation and frustration. The surgical stockings that you wear to keep down the swelling in your legs and aid circulation may cause your leg to itch along the whole incision. With them on, your legs feel hot and uncomfortable. In my case, I disliked wearing them so much that every time I lay down on the couch, I put my ankles up on one of the arms and took the stockings off.

The leg incision is more troublesome than the chest incision. The chest incision is uncomfortable for a few weeks, but the leg hurts, stings, and itches for months. It even hurts years later when you stoop down or squat on your haunches, such as when you change a tire on a car.

The chest incision also gets to itching, but it is never the nuisance that your leg is. The leg incision hits you periodically with a sharp pain like a needle every day or so. It lasts only a minute or two. Sometimes it's more frequent. Both of my legs still tingle and twitch at times, possibly from poor circulation. When this happens, it's almost impossible to sit still, and the only way to help is to take an aspirin or get up and walk, which can be embarrassing with company or in an office.

From the day you go the hospital, the nurses keep warning you not to cross your legs. Once the vein is removed from your leg, crossing them is forbidden. I haven't always observed this rule, and my lapses may be contributing to my nervous legs.

After five months, I still have considerable numbness along the area of my leg where the vein was removed. The other leg has a little numbness, but it is hardly noticeable. The tingling sensation, the itching, and the sharp little needle points are also missing from this leg. I presume I had them once, but I do not remember them as much. Hence, I assume these irritations will pass with time in the leg that was just operated on.

The greatest numbness is felt in the left side of my chest, where the mammary artery was removed. This seems to be diminishing rapidly and may soon be gone.

In the early days after the operation, the wounds are purple in appearance. This deep shade gradually changes to red and then to pink, becoming normal in a few months. When I was on the ship, I was embarrassed and refused to wear shorts or a swimsuit because the purplish color was clearly visible at the incision lines. A month later, it had turned red. For a younger person, the transition may be quicker. My original incision, by comparison, is hardly visible without close scrutiny and has been that way for years.

Because of the weakness and the traumatic nature of the experience, anger and frustration are common emotions. They occur not just in the hospital, as I described earlier, but also persist at home for a while. These feelings are not limited to the patient; the family itself may tend to strike out at the apparent injustice of having its members' lives violently disrupted. Time alone is needed to release these tensions and return the family to its normal level of relaxation.

Your doctor should be called if there is any sign of infection in your incisions or if you experience fever, chills, increased fatigue, shortness of breath, swelling, rapid weight gain, or a change in the rhythm of your heart, any of which may be a sign of a serious problem.

It should be realized that the operation doesn't set aside the past. It's not a complete start-over, replacing a person of sixty by an eighteen-year-old. At best it enables us to turn the clock back a little, to cheat a little on Father Time. This, in addition to the reduction in pain and the increased activity level, justifies the operation.

Obviously, I'm far better off than I was. That's all that any of us had hoped for. That's what I got. The immediate threat of disaster stands farther down the road. The Old Apparition has given me one more extension.

These, then, are the hopes and problems you face during your first weeks at home. In many respects, you are starting a new life.

13

A NEW LIFE
AND
A NEW SCHEDULE

In general, open heart surgery may have little effect on your previous pattern of life, other than to recapture what was lost. Sedentary workers usually return to work in four to six weeks. A friend of mine, Lowell Chrisman, who is a publisher for a magazine, had open heart bypass surgery on April 1, three months after mine, and on May 10 he began driving to work daily between Akron and Cleveland. To be sure, he worked only half a day in the beginning. During his second week of work, we met for lunch at a restaurant on his way home. He was full of energy and was thoroughly enjoying himself. He said, "I haven't felt so good in years!" This is a common expression of most persons who have gone through the operation.

Like myself, Lowell Chrisman was active almost immediately after arriving home. He had visitors from his office coming to his home daily, from the first week on. He interviewed and hired a new editor in his home the second week after the operation. The candidate flew in from out of town to be interviewed.

Lowell was fifty-three when he had his operation. His bypass was preceded by two heart attacks, the first of which had occurred three years earlier on a trip to Texas. He suffered some heart damage and was held in a Texas hospital until it was safe to travel. He flew home. His Akron doctor put him on a walking regimen, like the one I described earlier, and he was doing very well until the second attack. This second attack was quite severe, and he was lucky to have survived. When they advised bypass surgery for him, I asked him what his reaction was. "Wonderful," he said. "I looked forward to the operation. Why shouldn't I?" For him it opened up a whole new future after a very frightening experience.

I had not seen Lowell since before my own operation, and it is probable that I would not have learned of his experience had it not been for a strange set of coincidences, the kind of stuff movies delight in but which are rarely convincing and usually dull.

It all began on board the good ship *Rotterdam*. Here, another man from Akron and myself, and our families, were assigned to the same lifeboat. Considering that there were 952 passengers on board, this alone was a welcome surprise. That we even got to talking to each other during the lifeboat drill, with 120 passengers assigned to our boat, was also unlikely. But that he should mention by name only one person in Akron, a city of 260,000, who was a close personal friend of both of ours is stretching coincidence to the limit. No movie could get away with it. So you don't have to believe it either, even if it's true. Naturally, he mentioned the publisher friend when he found out I had written a book, which helped key the thing in.

I called Lowell as soon as we got home and found out he had just been home two weeks. Three weeks later we were having lunch together.

From some of my remarks, you may get the impression that only executives and white-collar workers can enjoy this type of operation, that it's reserved for a special breed of people. But unlike women, who seem to be above these problems to a large extent, blue-collar workers also qualify regularly for the experience.

They may not be as well represented in the hospitals as some of the other groups, but that's only because they work harder and keep in better shape than many of us.

Naturally, patients who perform heavy work need more time to prepare themselves for returning to work. Some who are less fortunate may have to find work of a less demanding nature. The state vocational rehabilitation center can often be of help in this regard.

While you're waiting to go back to work, what kind of a routine should you normally keep at home? Naturally, you can't just lie around and be waited on. As I pointed out, these tendencies catch up with you pretty quickly, and then you're in trouble.

The best way to prolong the pleasures as long as possible is to go through the motions of recovery.

This means you have to get up at a reasonable hour. I

tried sleeping in until 1 o'clock and having breakfast in bed, but I couldn't stand it. I got up between 7 and 8 every morning. In fact, if I overslept, my wife came up to the bedroom to see if I was still alive. She acted so frightened, I never tried it again. Mark up a round for my wife.

You should take a bath or shower regularly, too—as much for your friends as for yourself. At first you run the shower on your back so it won't hit your chest. You let it trickle over your shoulders onto your chest and pretend to wash it. Gradually you find it doesn't hurt at all, and you end up taking a complete shower. At first you can't breathe very deeply, so that your whistling and singing sound more like a gasp than a melody. But gradually you get your wind, in a few weeks, and pretty soon the whole house rocks to your merry melodies. The family knows you're recovering, and they wish you were back in the hospital so they could sleep.

You must always get dressed in street clothes. Get out of those pajamas. If you keep them on, you'll want to sleep all day long because it's psychological. Besides, they make it look like you're trying to get sympathy, and you must create the opposite impression. That way you'll get it without asking.

At first you should take a rest every morning and afternoon. Mine usually lasted until lunch, at which time I took a break to eat and then came back and watched TV from the couch.

I always walked religiously every day. Starting with the second day I got home, my wife drove me to the mall. Cold weather and very hot humid weather still bother me, so I have found the mall the best means for avoiding both. Extremes of temperature are taxing on the heart because they force the body to work harder. They should be avoided when exercising.

My first day out, I made only a half trip around the mall. In a few days I made a complete cycle. And in a couple of weeks I was making six laps, about three miles.

When I got home, I was so tired, I lay down and slept. Walking, I understand, is one of the healthiest exercises you can do when you have heart problems. It helps the circulation and strengthens the heart.

One pamphlet I read also suggested doing light work

around the house, such as helping with the dishes, but these kinds of comments should not be taken too seriously. They can have lingering results and should not be mentioned in any set of notes worth serious consideration. I did the dishes on several occasions during my convalescence, because I wanted something to do, and I actually enjoyed it. It was only with a great deal of effort and willpower that I was able to break myself of the habit. My wife still thinks I ought to help more often, and I don't know how long it's going to take to get her retrained.

Believe me, convalescence is not the time to be weak-kneed and pusillanimous. It's not the time to let feelings of gratitude and affection warp your judgment. You must maintain the equilibrium established in the battle of the sexes. You owe this much to your compatriots and the fellow heart patients who will follow in your noble footsteps.

If you really feel a need to express your gratitude to those who have given so much of themselves to help you, try taking them out to dinner or the theater. Even if they end up paying, keep in mind it's the thought that counts.

Church is also a good place to go, and if you can control your urge to be thankful and hold yourself in check when they pass the collection plate, you can get by for very little—and still get the benefits. I always give a little bit more because my wife has a very sharp elbow. Since my operation, I've been little more than a Pavlovian dog, as you can see. In fact, if you should visit my home and catch me doing the dishes, you'll know that I do not speak in jest. Even my sixteen-year-old son is stronger than I. How I long once more for the good old days when I first came home!

But alas, those days are gone forever, unless I should return perchance for *thirds!* What an unfortunate set of choices!

CONCLUDING REMARKS

It's difficult to see how you can take 180 pages or so to write a book and then summarize the whole thing in three. There's something almost larcenous about the very idea.

Nevertheless, let me do it, as a gesture of my concern for your well-being.

Everyone who's had heart surgery has a right to live to a ripe old age. To enhance these chances, and to increase your peace of mind, you need to consider the following things:

1. The purpose of coronary artery bypass graft surgery, or other types of surgery, is to restore you to an active, full life. When you get out of the hospital and you feel lousy and down-in-the-dumps, remember that you will soon feel better than you've felt for years.

2. Returning to gainful employment takes time and sometimes requires adjustments, but once you achieve a renewed confidence and sense of well-being, you'll soon appreciate how lucky you are, compared to so many others in the world with far worse debilitations.

3. You owe it to yourself and those dependent on you to reduce the risk factors involved in heart attacks. You should quit smoking, keep your blood pressure under control, keep your weight down, and follow a diet that is low in salt, saturated fats, and cholesterol.

4. Avoid stress-producing situations that are self-imposed and usually unnecessary. These include situations where you put yourself under pressure by setting excessively tight deadlines and worrying about time schedules. I used to delight in situations in which one activity would follow upon another like clockwork. It was fun to get many things done in sequence under tight drill, like an army lock step. But when things went wrong and delays set in, I would become extremely impatient and frustrated.

   Today, when I leave for the airport, I add half an hour to the time I tell myself I need. The extra time at the airport I use to walk the long corridors, substituting them for the mall. I almost never sandwich two meetings back to back, so if one runs overtime, I avoid the pressure of wanting to leave and being forced to stay.

5. Situations that anger you should be avoided. If you encounter frustrations, try to resolve them quickly and

amicably. To help me here, I took a page from the letters of Benjamin Franklin. Every time I get very angry, I mark the day on the calendar with a big X. Those big Xs can be very embarrassing when you realize they represent a lack of self-control. You won't believe the effect this has had on my life, let alone on those whom I love. Today's calendar has fewer than one tenth of the markings I used to give myself two years ago—and I've become a tougher grader, too.

6. As your recovery progresses, you will be able to appreciate more fully the miracle of the surgery you have just had. The increased blood flow through your arteries should mean less angina, perhaps none at all. Since my second operation, over a period of five months, I have taken exactly one nitroglycerin tablet. This compares with five or more a day before. Even that one may have been unnecessary. I was having a pain that may have been caused by the operation, but I wondered if it might be angina.

7. You will probably be able to sustain physical activity and exercise with a much greater capacity than before. You almost certainly will be able to take up activities such as golf and hiking that were out of the question before. In sum, you are going to feel better than you have ever felt for a long, long time, and you will probably live longer as well.

Perhaps my most heartening and tender experience occurred in an interview I had with a wonderful, brave woman at the clinic. She was fifty-seven when I met her. She had had a long, sad history of heart problems. Her first heart attack occurred when she was forty-one. She recovered from that one and was doing fairly well until another attack struck her down six years later. From then on her problems worsened. Angina became a constant companion, and she became a total invalid. She was suffering from pulmonary edema (water in the lungs) and congestive heart failure. Shortly after her second attack, her husband died of a heart attack, and one of her children died. (One son is still living.)

After her husband's death, she spent most of her time in the hospital and was kept on oxygen when she was home. Her condition and angina pain were so intense that she was almost entirely restricted to bed or a wheelchair. In the early days she could still drive a car on occasion, depending on the angina.

She was a devout Christian; although she lived only 200 feet from the church, she was unable to make it to the services.

The year before I met her, her doctors put her on nitro paste (the paste they tape to your leg, as a supplement to nitroglycerin pills). This newly developed drug was truly a miracle drug for her: It enabled her for the first time in years to walk about in her own home.

She had heard of bypass surgery, but her doctors had discouraged it, feeling she would not survive in her poor condition. But the new technology developed in the field encouraged her to try. On May 4, ten years after her second heart attack, they operated, performing several bypasses and a heart-valve repair.

When I met her, she was sitting up, eating lunch. She got up afterwards and walked around the halls. She made this trip several times a day.

She was a pleasant, gentle person with a kind manner. Her voice was weak but cheerful. She was going home on May 19, two weeks after the operation. The trip to her home in southern Ohio would be by ambulance, but she looked forward to it. She became tired as we talked and had to rest, and I was struck by her morale and hopefulness, which were never crushed by those long years of suffering.

After the operation, she required almost no nitroglycerin. She was no longer on nitro paste, and her other medication had been reduced.

I met her later in the hall, as she was out walking. She smiled as I came up and we talked for a few minutes. She was returning from class—the same one I had attended a few months earlier (where the patient had fainted). She knew of my operation and could see the results of what could be accomplished.

"Do you think I will be all right?" she asked. I nodded.

"They haven't been lying to me, have they?" I assured her they wouldn't do that. As I left her, she seemed very pleased and walked slowly to her room.

I watched her as she moved out of sight. A sense of pride and compassion swept over me. Even though I was just a visitor, I sensed how doctors must feel at times when they are right and see the results of their efforts. All the sad times and moments of despair are made worthwhile by each success— each grateful patient, each life restored.

What more is there to say, or hope for?

I close by wishing you my very best, and I sincerely hope you return from your operation with as much luck and appreciation for what has been accomplished as I have. I look outside and see the trees and hear the birds and never appreciated them more. Like a child, I am seeing them for the first time.

May God go with you.

APPENDIX

Here is an association you might like to join:

The Mended Hearts, Inc.
7320 Greenville Avenue
Dallas, TX 75231

There are numerous local chapters made up of people like ourselves.

Another group that strikes me as being very interesting is the

Fraternity of Recouped Hearts
Box 7163
Arlington, VA 22207

This second group provides a regular newsletter and sponsors many things of interest to heart patients and their families, including a special lapel pin to help us spot our "blood" brothers in a crowd.

INDEX